Shampoo-Free

Shampoo-Free

A DIY Guide to Putting Down the Bottle
and Embracing Healthier, Happier Hair

Savannah Born

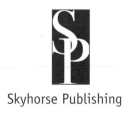

Skyhorse Publishing

Skyhorse Publishing books may be purchased in bulk at special discounts for sales promotion, corporate gifts, fund-raising, or educational purposes. Special editions can also be created to specifications. For details, contact the Special Sales Department, Skyhorse Publishing, 307 West 36th Street, 11th Floor, New York, NY 10018 or info@skyhorsepublishing.com.

Skyhorse® and Skyhorse Publishing® are registered trademarks of Skyhorse Publishing, Inc.®, a Delaware corporation.

Visit our website at www.skyhorsepublishing.com.

10 9 8 7 6 5 4 3 2 1

Library of Congress Cataloging-in-Publication Data is available on file.

Cover design by Sarah Brody
Cover photo credit Thinkstock

Original photos by Sarah Grieb and Erin Albrecht

Print ISBN: 978-1-63220-632-9
Ebook ISBN: 978-1-63220-778-4

Printed in China

Shampoo-Free

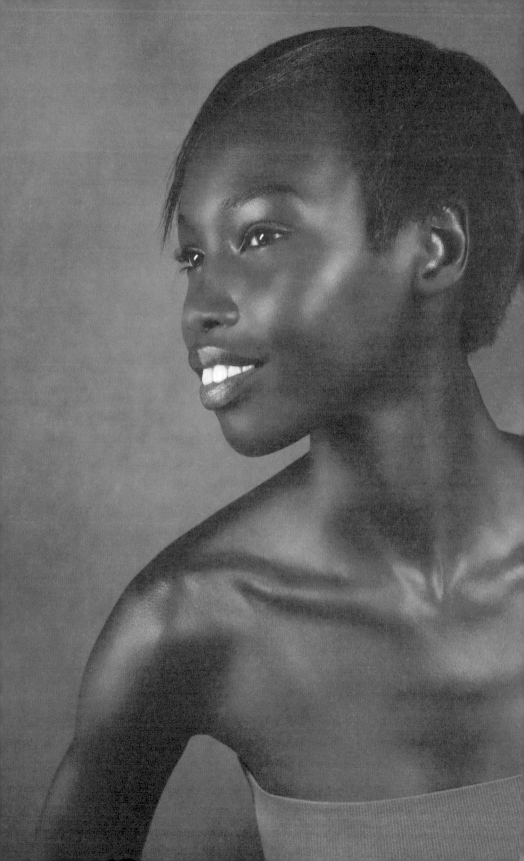

Contents

Introduction

Imagine a life without shampoo . . . Whether your reaction is "ew!" or "woo-hoo!" the idea is intriguing, no?

Perhaps you've heard whispers of "no poo" at a social gathering. Were your friends frankly discussing their digestive habits? More likely they were talking about a health-and-beauty trend that's taking the beauty world by storm. Going "no poo," aka shampoo-free, has gotten press from outlets like *the New York Times*, *Elle*, and *Marie Claire*. A quick Google search shows the practice blowing up all over the health, beauty, and DIY blogosphere. Growing ranks of celebrities are cutting way back on—or even ditching—shampoo, or incorporating shampoo alternatives into their hair routine. (Catherine Zeta-Jones uses beer!)

A shampoo-free lifestyle is not only possible, it's filled with benefits. Would you like to stop spending so much money on hair care? Would you prefer to live without words you can't pronounce cluttering the labels of your beauty products? Is your hair lackluster? Do you find yourself needing to shampoo it every single day—and would you like a break from that? Do you want soft, fluffy, shiny, healthy, gorgeous locks?

If you've said yes to any of these questions, this book's for you. A life without the endless cycle of lather, rinse, repeat is within your reach, and can actually help your hair look and feel better than ever.

While I enjoy the playful ambiguity of "no poo"—the common moniker for the movement—the phrase "no sham" is equally as fun, and just as fitting. Because that's exactly what the shampoo-free set wants to leave behind: the falseness of the ingredients, the lie that we *need* a product to clean our hair when that product didn't even exist until very recently.

Why not ditch the sham, ditch the poo, and find what works for you? This book is your one-stop guide to living a life free of shampoo. If you can't bear the thought of dumping shampoo completely, check out the section on "low poo" alternatives, which provide the benefits of shampoos without the harsh chemicals or unnecessary add-ons. Whatever method you choose, healthier, happier hair is on the horizon. This book covers the whys and the hows, the ins and outs, and the ups and the downs of eliminating shampoo from your routine. You'll hear from folks who've successfully made the transition, why they're glad they did so, and their tips to help you succeed. Welcome to Shampoo Freedom!

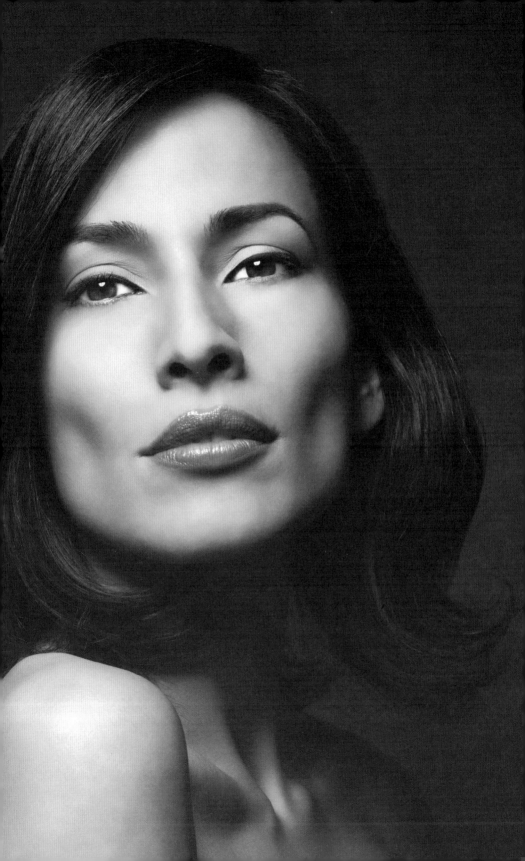

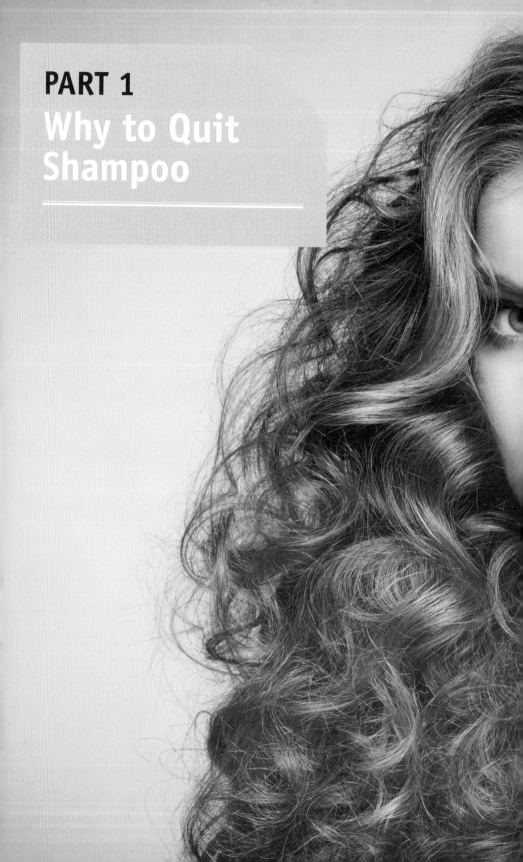

PART 1
Why to Quit
Shampoo

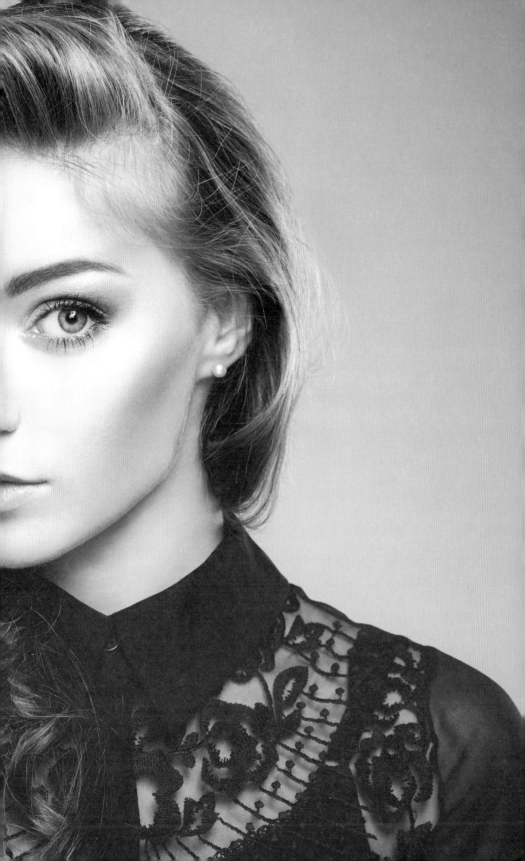

People have had hair for far longer than shampoo has been around to clean hair. Of course, many things we have today I wouldn't wish to live without (antibiotics, contact lenses, on-demand video streaming), but that doesn't mean that taking steps to simplify our health and beauty routines lacks merit. Chemicals have improved modern life and the human body in many ways, but irresponsible human use of chemicals has its consequences too (think cancer; think climate change).

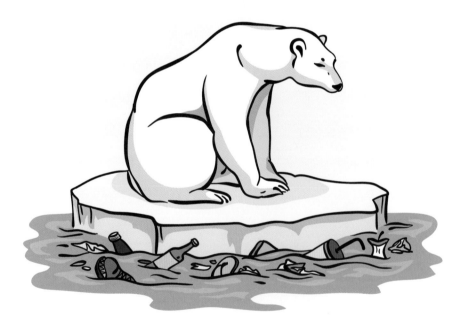

This book is not meant to give the impression that "chemical" is a dirty word—every substance is chemical! Baking soda is just as "chemical" as polyoxyethylene; even water is "chemical." And "natural" products are not necessarily better, or even danger-free. Poison ivy comes direct from Mother Earth; that doesn't mean you want it in your favorite hand cream. But chemicals can and do affect our health and our ecosystem, and not always for the best. Some of the commonly used chemicals in our everyday beauty products may be worth avoiding. Particularly if they're unnecessary and have easy, suitable, cost-effective alternatives, why not eliminate them? Minimizing the multisyllabic ingredients in our lives seems more likely to prove beneficial than harmful, don't you think?

In the case of shampoo, a little research and a bit of practice show that there's no need for sodium lauryl sulfates and the parabens contained in nearly all common shampoo brands. Certain shampoo ingredients may even be harmful to our health or the ecosystem's. Before we delve into the details of these ingredients, we'll learn how shampoo came to be a staple in our daily lives.

The History of Sham-poo

Shampoo as we know it now did not exist until very recently. Historically, people cleaned their hair using ash, animal fat, or vegetable starch and used perfume or essential oils to condition it and add fragrance, as well as tools to scrape away gunk and grime—it's a far cry from the sudsy wet lather and quick rinses we are familiar with today.

The first manufactured shampoo didn't appear on the market until the early 1900s, and the types of shampoos we use today not until the 1970s. We can trace the roots of modern shampoo,

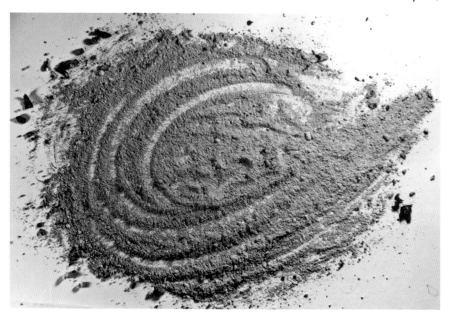

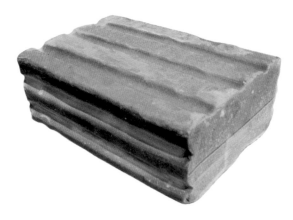

however, back to the 1700s. The English word "shampoo" comes from the Hindi *chāmpo*, which refers to the Indian custom of massaging the body, including the head and the hair, using herbs and plants for cleansing.

During colonial times, Europeans in India grew fond of *chāmpo*, and the practice subsequently became popular in Europe. The word "shampoo" came to describe specifically head and scalp massaging, and later the word shampoo was coopted from this massaging practice to refer to the cleaning substance rubbed into the scalp, rather than just the rubbing itself. The verb "shampoo" as we use it dates back to around 1860, and the noun referring to the cleansing substance to a few years later.

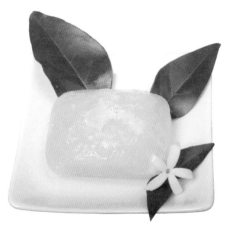

European proto-shampoos were made by putting bits of soap and maybe an herb or two into water. They left a lot to be desired. When soap was used, it interacted with hard water and left a scummy residue, not to mention that it was harsh on the eyes. In stepped chemists with their bag of scientific tricks to improve upon this formula. Shampooing habits were radically different from today's for most of the twentieth century. In 1908, the *New York Times* published an article reassuring readers that it was okay to shampoo once every two weeks rather than the currently

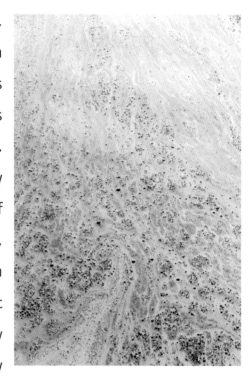

conventional once a month, although according to "several hair specialists," says the *Times*, "from a month to six weeks should be a better interval if the hair is in fairly good condition." Apparently, "Every woman likes to have her hair not only daintily and becomingly arranged but soft and glossy in appearance and texture." I wouldn't generalize quite so broadly, but for many ladies a fine hairdo is still on trend a century-plus later.

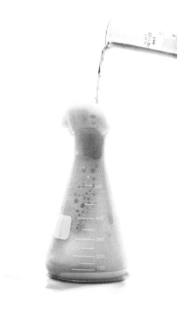

The antique habit of brushing your hair one hundred strokes a day makes sense

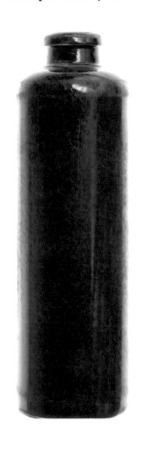

in light of this minimal shampooing. Hair brushing would help distribute the scalp's natural oils and reduce gunky buildup. The first commercially available shampoos hit shelves in the 1930s, with Dr. John Breck generally credited as being the first to offer bottled shampoo. Breck shampoo was only sold in salons until the mid-1940s. Is it hard to believe that before then, there were no at-home shampoo bottles? What about that the formula of these proto-modern shampoos was typically so strong hair was washed only once a week?

If the name Breck sounds familiar, it's because of the Breck Girl ads: Softly lit faces and flowing locks set against soft pastel backgrounds adorned the glossy pages of popular women's magazines from the 1930s through the 1970s. Breck shampoo was available in three formulas—for dry hair, for oily hair, and for normal hair—because "every woman is different," though you wouldn't think so from looking at the ads, which suffered from a serious lack of diversity, chromatic or otherwise.

Nearly all of the ads show eerily similar button noses dotting pale complexions framed by waves of almost-always blond hair.

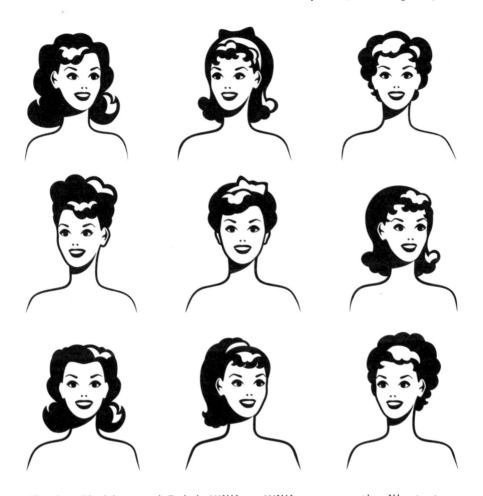

Charles Sheldon and Ralph William Williams were the illustrators who created the portraits of the Breck girls. Sheldon created 107 iconic portraits, and Williams was responsible for transitioning to employing celebrities and professional models, rather than the so-called everywoman seen in previous ads. The Archives Center at the Smithsonian Institution has a collection of nearly 220 "original artwork pieces" related to the Breck ad campaigns, most of which are Breck Girl portraits. Famous Breck Girls (actually, they were *women*, but that's a discussion for another book) included

Cybill Shepherd, Jaclyn Smith, Kim Basinger, Brooke Shields, Farrah Fawcett, and Christie Brinkley. The Breck Girls signaled a cultural shift in hair habits: They popularized daily at-home shampooing.

Farrah Fawcett and Christie Brinkley form an interesting link. In the 1970s, when daily shampooing first became popular, popular television commercials from Faberge and Prell broadcast live action shots of Farrah Fawcett's bouncing locks or Christie Brinkley's shiny mane, and attributed the lovely luster to daily shampooing. This too can be yours, promise the ads. (They are available on YouTube—and the folly of advertising seems extra clear when it's flavored with the singular aesthetic of a long-past decade.) Thanks to these commercials, daily shampooing was recast as healthy and best for hair. Of course, if we're to believe the "lather, rinse, repeat" mantra, we'll be essentially trapped in a never-ending shampoo loop, an infinite shower. But that didn't stop the cultural consensus from morphing to consider less-than-daily shampooing as gross.

Realizing that the shampoos we use today—and the practice of daily shampooing—have only been in existence for a few decades shines a light on how unnecessary they are. Who stood to gain from wide adoption of the notion that hair without daily cleansing becomes filthy and decidedly un-Farrah-esque? Advertisers jumped on the chance to sell us a product we didn't really need. They told us what hair was supposed to look like, and they promised they could make ours fit the mold. This alone feels like a reason to reexamine habitual shampoo use. But if you still aren't sure that you want to abandon the shampoos you're used to, read on to learn about other reasons to relinquish the habit.

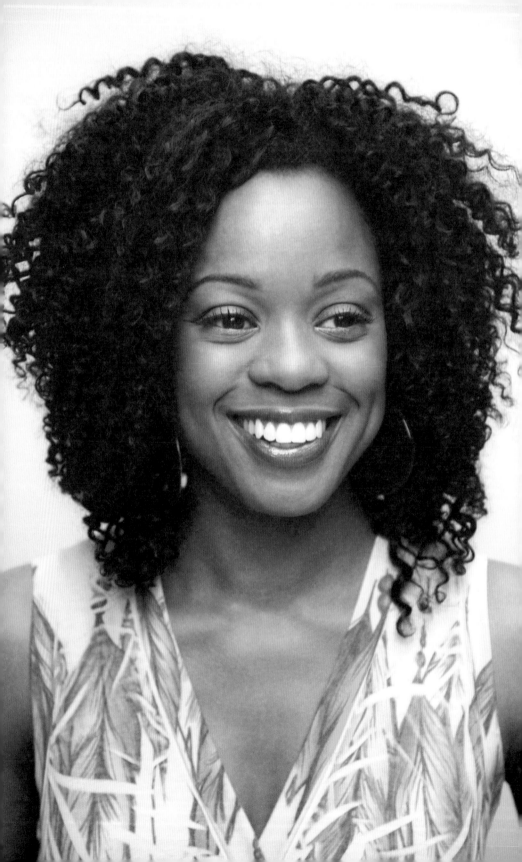

Don't Needs, Don't Wants

Now let's turn to the most compelling reasons to leave that shampoo bottle behind.

First of all, we just don't need it that much! We've essentially been duped by shampoo manufacturers and advertisers into thinking that we must use shampoo more often than we actually must. (In fact, there is no "must.") Nearly any dermatologist you ask will say, "Less is more." Secondly, even if we're using it less often, shampoo may contain some gunk better off left behind

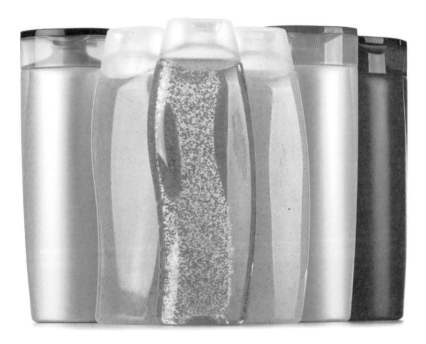

entirely. The common ingredients in most popular shampoo brands are mostly a bundle of things we might not need or want.

Your classic drugstore shampoo concoction will typically contain a few key elements: a detergent to clean (like sodium lauryl sulfate); ingredients to improve its texture and appearance, by, for example, making it thick or foamy (polyethylene glycol is one); preservatives to keep it stable (usually parabens); a conditioner to soften hair after the detergent has left it stripped (like dimethicone); and any handful of other additives, like fragrances, coloring, and so on. Specialty shampoos, such as dandruff shampoos, will contain other ingredients as well as the typical ones. Some of these substances are perfectly innocuous, but many are unnecessary and a few are downright dangerous. Let's see what that inscrutable list of ingredients really tells us.

The Problems with Poo

What potential problems come with the medleys inside our shampoo bottles? Let's tackle the most serious first: health and environmental risks. Any extreme claims about the dangers of shampoo are probably unfounded. If you've seen a chain email about sodium lauryl sulfate causing cancer, approach with caution.

It's good to be as wary of broad claims about ingredients causing extreme health problems as it is to be wary of product manufacturers who care most about the bottom line, to the possible exclusion of 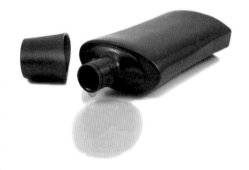 the health, safety, and satisfaction of customers and the planet. In each case, consider the evidence. It's always good to ask, who is making this claim and why, what are the sources, and what might it harm or help to believe? If it sounds like (or is) a chain email, chances are it's not evidence-based or well founded.

That said, consumer safety groups and agencies (like the FDA and the EWG) exist to help us evaluate the ingredients in the products we use and consume. So what does the research say about which everyday shampoo ingredients might be a problem?

SULFATES

We'll start with the big boys—the much-maligned sodium lauryl sulfate, and its ilk: ammonium lauryl sulfate, sodium laureth sulfate, sodium lauryl ether sulfate, and basically any other ingredient you read with the word "sulfate" in it. These are the detergents, the grease strippers. They are strong and mighty, binding to grease *and* to water, thus enabling the grease to be captured then washed away. They're also one source of that delightful foam a classic shampoo entails. But are they bad for you? Well, yes, no, and maybe so. Frantic claims that sodium lauryl sulfate causes cancer are not supported by any evidence. Major agencies that determine whether substances are carcinogenic, including OSHA and the International Agency for Research on Cancer, maintain that SLS poses no cancer threat. The American Cancer Society is also quick to refute the notion that SLS is linked to cancer. The Environmental Working Group rates SLS a "low hazard" based on "fair" data.

SLS does carry some risks though: It can cause skin irritation if you have sensitive skin or leave it on too long. This irritant property is why shampoo stings when it gets in your eyes. It's also good to steer clear of eating SLS. (Hopefully not a problem for you with shampoo?—but note that it's one of the reasons your toothpaste tube warns against swallowing what you brush with, as most toothpaste also contains SLS.) If you just can't break away from your delicious toothpaste-and-shampoo diet and you end up eating too much SLS, you'll get the runs. Diarrhea is a far cry from cancer, but still unpleasant.

Another consideration when it comes to SLS is its impact on the environment. According to Environment Canada's Domestic Substance List, SLS is likely to be an environmental toxin—which alone could be reason enough to stay 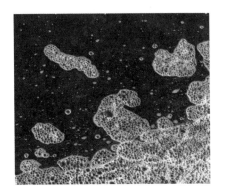 away from it, considering how much we wash down the drain each day with our ferocious shampooing. And a study by the National Institute of Health suggests that some shampoo detergents washed down the drain destroy the algae that serve as a nutrient source for other aquatic organisms.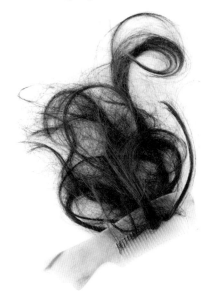

There's also concern about how SLS interacts with hair itself. According to certain doctors (and many successfully shampoo-free folks), using SLS daily can be problematic for hair, gradually stripping the oils in hair that maintain its health, and degrading the hair's protein structures— with the end result of interfering with hair growth.

The verdict is still out on just how bad SLS is for us, our hair, or where it goes when we wash it down the drain. It may be fine. But if so, why all the cancer claims? That may have something to do with sodium laureth sulfate: a slightly different spelling—and a different chemical makeup—from sodium lauryl sulfate. Sodium laureth sulfate (SLES) is created when sodium lauryl sulfate (SLS) undergoes the process of ethoxylation (that's what the "eth" distinguishing "laureth" from "lauryl" refers to), which is done to make the chemical less irritating. SLES does have some potential to be problematic because of the byproducts it may result in. See below on 1,4-dioxane and ethylene oxide for more details. SLS and SLES, which are both created from coconut oil (so natural!), are made

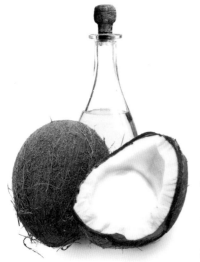

up of molecules small enough to enter the body through topical application— another reason to double-consider any possible risk.

POLYETHYLENE GLYCOL

This ethylene oxide polymer's dissolving power helps clean the hair (and there's a chance it's dissolving more than it should, stripping hair of proteins, taking the good along with the bad). But, like sodium laureth sulfate, its real problem is 1,4-dioxane, caused by ethylene oxide.

ETHYLENE OXIDE AND 1,4-DIOXANE

This is some seriously scary stuff. The chemical 1,4-dioxane is an impurity byproduct of the ethoxylation process—when the chemical ethylene oxide is added to petroleum products. The result is a foamier and reportedly less irritating product. There's no requirement to list 1,4-dioxane on labels—in fact, because it is a byproduct, you'll never see it listed directly. Instead, you have to look out for the ingredients that may result in the impurity. In addition to sodium laureth sulfate, keep a look out for sodium myreth sulfate and any ingredients containing the syllables "xynol," "ceteareth," and "oleth" or the prefix "PEG" (these are polyethylene glycol blends), as these manufactured compounds may have brought their nasty friend 1,4-dioxane to the party.

What's so bad about 1,4-dioxane? The FDA and the EPA list it as a probable human carcinogen, and 1,4-dioxane molecules, because of their small size, can readily penetrate human skin and be absorbed into the body. What's worse, 1,4-dioxane is an easy chemical for product manufacturers to remove, but most often, they don't bother (in one study, a series of tests found levels of 1,4-dioxane in a good number of common products). It can also be toxic to our internal organs and is particularly dangerous for young people or pregnant women (well, the young people they are carrying). In Canada—our progressive northern sister with its magical universal health care—1,4-dioxane is officially banned from consumer products. United States manufacturers assure us that low levels mean we won't see any resulting health issues. Yet even if the levels are very low, it's not known if or how they might add up over time. Ethylene oxide itself (which creates the 1,4-dioxane impurity) doesn't get a clean bill either—it's also a known carcinogen.

ETHANOLAMINES

Alas, 1,4-dioxane isn't the only cancer concern. Ethanolamines, such as monoethanolamine (MEA), diethanolamine (DEA), and triethanolamine (TEA), or any variation thereof (cocamide DEA, lauramide DEA, linoleamide MEA—and plenty more), are a protein-and-alcohol combination that works to emulsify, perfume, or adjust the pH of consumer products ranging from shampoo to makeup to floor cleaner.

The big issue with these is that when they are present in a product that also contains nitrogen-producing preservatives, they may interact and result in nitrosamines—another nasty byproduct. All nitrosamines (over a dozen exist) are either known to be or considered likely to be carcinogenic.

Animal and human studies indicate an alarming array of problems stemming from nitrosamines. They have been demonstrated to cause several types of cancer in rats, hamsters, and mice. They are toxic to organs, in particular the liver and kidneys, interfere with the reproductive abilities of human sperm, and possibly impede proper brain development in fetuses when the mother is exposed. They also bioaccumulate, meaning they remain on the skin, particularly when used in hair dyes, lotions, and yes, *shampoo*, giving them an extra opportunity to do their dirty work.

DEA is enough of a potential hazard to be banned from use in European cosmetics due to safety concerns. In California, a lawsuit was recently filed against manufacturers of products containing cocamide DEA. Luckily, it's pretty easy to avoid nitrosamines—just stay away from anything with DEA, TEA, or MEA in the ingredients list.

PARABENS

Another contested ingredient, parabens are used to preserve and stabilize products, eliminating bacteria and fungus. Parabens are another great example of why the words "chemical" and "natural" don't always mean what product package design would have us believe. Parabens are made from plants, so they must be totally fine for us, right? Don't be too quick to assume that. What does the research say?

Parabens have been found in breast cancer tumors. That sounds alarming, but correlation doesn't equal causation: No evidence actually suggests that the parabens found in tumors contributed to the cancer. In fact, parabens are present within most Americans' bodies, according to investigation from the CDC (kind of scary, but most of us don't have breast cancer). The general opinion among researchers is that the paraben level in most of your beauty products isn't high enough to cause any problems. That said, some scientists have expressed concerns over parabens, in particular that they may be linked to early-onset puberty in girls because of their estrogen-mimicking properties. If you'd rather not take the chance, watch out in particular for butyl-, isobutyl-, propyl-, and isopropyl parabens—these long-chain parabens may be particularly problematic.

If you are using a cosmetic product that will spoil without some kind of preservative, alternatives that don't present the same concerns, such as vitamins C or E, are a good option.

METHYLISOTHIAZOLINONE

Methylisothiazolinone is another type of preservative the cautious consumer will want to keep away from. It is rated a moderate hazard based on limited data by the Environmental Working Group because it can cause allergic reactions and was shown to be toxic to mammal brain cells in laboratory studies. Originally, consumer safety guidelines suggested that as long as manufacturers kept levels below 100 ppm (parts per million), all was safe. But a new report from the European Commission's Scientific Committee on Consumer Safety calls for more caution after further evaluating methylisothiazolinone's effects on consumers: "Current clinical data indicate that 100 ppm MI in cosmetic products is not safe for the consumer." This is especially true in leave-on (rather than rinse-off) products. Sounds like one to permanently bench.

FORMALDEHYDE

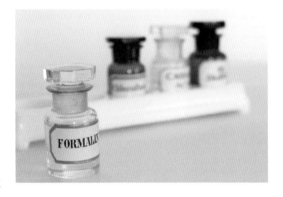

Apart from seeming straight-up gross thanks to its association with embalming and preserving dead stuff, formaldehyde is another problem ingredient to look out for. Yes, in addition to keeping cadavers fresh, formaldehyde is sometimes found in health and beauty products, where it is added to prevent the growth of microorganisms. It also makes hair become stiff and as a result is particularly common in hair-straightening chemicals.

But besides the ick factor, is it dangerous? Definitely. It's another known carcinogen. It's also neurotoxic, and it leads to asthma symptoms and allergic reactions, if you want to pick your poison. Manufacturers are held to strictly regulated standards to ensure that the levels of formaldehyde added to shampoo are safe.

But hair-care professionals who are repeatedly exposed to the chemical might be at increased risk. All things considered, it's a good one to skip.

It's not just the word "formaldehyde" you need to check the label for if you want to avoid it. Certain other chemical preservatives release small amounts of formaldehyde over time, to keep the antiseptic action going. These include: DMDM hydantoin, diazolidinyl urea, imidazolidinyl urea, quaternium-15, Bronopol, and sodium hydroxymethylglycinate.

PHTHALATES

Phthalates, such as dibutyl phthalate, dimethyl phthalate, diethyl phthalate (or anything with "phthalate" in the name), or butyl ester, are also sometimes known as "plasticizers"; they increase the flexible plasticity of certain materials. They also

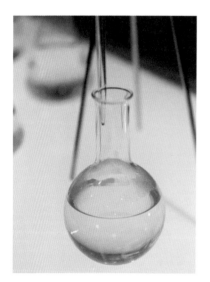

have solvent properties, and are used in a wide range of products, from raingear to flooring to shampoo. The issue with phthalates is that they may interfere with hormone levels. The FDA says there isn't a conclusive risk (at least, there's not enough information to suggest one yet), but more studies are demonstrating a possible link between phthalate exposure and developmental abnormalities in the reproductive systems of male fetuses.

Evidence also exists that the phthalates in baby products (like plastic toys or baby soaps and shampoos) may wind up inside the baby's body and cause problems that way. Biomonitoring by the CDC detected the presence of phthalates in the general U.S. population, indicating that exposure to phthalates is "widespread"; the CDC calls for further research on the health impacts of phthalate exposure.

"FRAGRANCE"

One of the potentially worst ingredients is one that sounds the least scary. Did you know that anything can be added to a product as a fragrance because there is no requirement to disclose what fragrance ingredients actually are? The aforementioned phthalates can 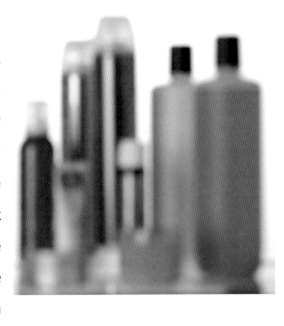 be present in fragrance blends, but there's no way for us to know by reading the label. One study evaluating the chemicals present in fragrance blends found around fourteen each in nearly twenty different products—and not one was listed. In addition to their potential for hormone interference, fragrances tend to contain chemicals that cause allergic reaction. "Buy fragrance free wherever possible," says the EWG.

SPECIALTY SHAMPOOS

Shampoos formulated for special purposes can pose additional risks. Three in particular carry noteworthy hazards.

Dandruff Shampoos

There's been some evidence that fungicides from dandruff shampoos, such as antimycotic climbazole, are polluting our water supply, affecting animals and plants who depend on that water to survive. The plants that process our wastewater aren't quite good enough to filter out certain chemicals, including fungicides. (Remember those reports about the medley of pharmaceutical drugs found in drinking water?) This can impact a range of creatures, from water's tiniest residents, like algae, which are killed by even low concentrations of fungicides, to the larger creatures, like plants and fish, whose growth can be stunted by the chemicals.

There's also the issue of coal tar, which is commonly used in dandruff shampoos for its ability to relieve itchy, scaly skin. Coal tar applied to the scalp is meant to cause the top layer of dead scalp skin to shed and to slow new scalp skin growth. But coal tar (and ingredients that contain it, such as aminophenol, diaminobenzene, and phenylenediamine) is classified as a carcinogen by several agencies, and many coal tar products are not allowed in Europe. For what it's worth, the FDA does not ban coal tar from dandruff shampoos, but overexposure to it is risky.

Antibacterial Cleansers

Certain shampoos and other harsh cleansers may be linked to the rise of drug-resistant bacteria: specifically, antimicrobial products containing quaternary ammonium compounds. When they're washed down the drain and become diluted, it allows bacteria with a natural resistance to them to flourish and grow—and these same bacteria can then show resistance to antibiotic treatments. If these antimicrobials are in our water supply, they may be consumed by animals or used to grow plants that we eat, potentially leading to drug-resistant infections in humans.

Another antibacterial ingredient to watch out for is the chemical triclosan (liquid form) or triclocarban (solid form). In addition to its potential contribution to antibiotic resistance in bacteria, triclosan and triclocarban can harm the animals who live in the water supply they contaminate by interfering with thyroid and hormone levels. The chemical also enters the food chain at the aquatic level, where it can accumulate in fatty tissue (in fish we eat, and then in our own fat stores, for example). Pregnant and breastfeeding women are advised to stay away due to evidence that triclosan disrupts endocrine and thyroid function.

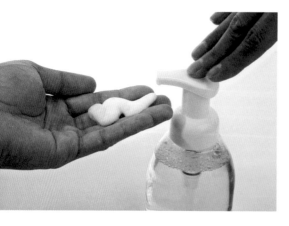

Antibacterial cleansers may sound like a good idea, but the FDA admits there's no evidence plain old soap and hot water aren't just as effective. And the FDA is now reviewing whether triclosan is safe to use at all; the case has been reopened based on growing evidence of potential problems. In general, antibacterial and antimicrobial ingredients seem to be more harmful than helpful. Keep them out of your household's shampoos, soaps, and toothpastes.

Microbeads

This advice goes for all products containing microbeads: Do not buy them. Often found in face washes and sometimes in shampoos, microbeads won't hurt you, but they will hurt the environment. When these plastic beads designed to provide extra exfoliating power are washed down the drain, they stay as plastic and beady as ever as they accumulate in our water system. They are causing terrible environmental damage to the Great Lakes, and the attorney general of New York is currently looking to ban them entirely. Get the same abrasive action from sea salt or brown sugar, with none of the nasty aftereffects.

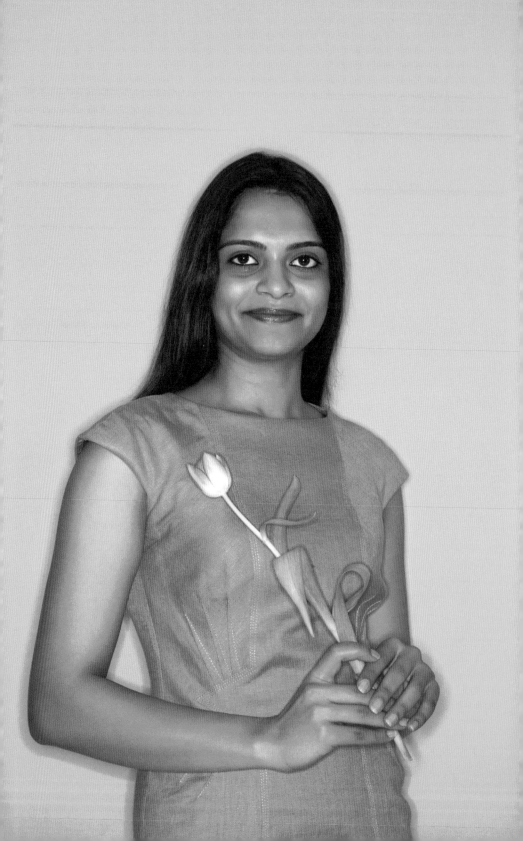

The Supporting Crew

That about does it for the real bad guys, but there are a few other considerations—or ingredients you may have heard to stay away from. Are those really worth avoiding?

ALCOHOL

Alcohol's not necessarily bad for you (you know, in moderation) or your hair, but it can dry hair out, especially if your hair is curly. Whether alcohol in your hair-care products might be a problem depends on what type of alcohol it is. Fatty alcohols provide a softening effect by attaching oil to water. The ones to stay away from, if alcohol dries your hair, are the short-chain alcohols, usually found in gels or hair sprays—though even then these may be formulated with fatty alcohols and present at low enough levels to counter any drying effect. But if your products are making your hair frizzy—particularly if you have curly hair—it's best to stay away from the short-chain alcohols. These include: SD alcohol, SD alcohol 40, Alcohol Denat, 1-Propanol, propyl alcohol, and isopropyl alcohol. Overall verdict? Know your alcohols, and proceed with caution.

SILICONE

Silicone-based smoothers, like dimethicone, are considered safe, and are popular in hair products (as well as other makeup and skin-care products) for their ability to impart instant sleekness and manageability. The potential problem with silicone is that while a little goes a long way, a lot can be too much. Overusing silicones may mean they accumulate on hair, preventing the strands from receiving oxygen and moisture. Silicone can protect your hair by coating it, but don't overdo it. Watch out for overuse of silicones—especially if they're in not just your shampoo or conditioner but your hair serums or other hair products as well. That would mean your hair never gets a break.

Used sparingly, silicone is a wonderful frizz tamper. It's helpful to learn about the different kinds of silicones to know which is best in which situation. There are water-soluble silicones, meaning water can remove them. If you are purely "no poo" or use a non-sulfate shampoo or are a co-washer, stick to water-soluble silicones. Dimethicone copolyol and cyclomethicone are good options for the shampoo-free set. They evaporate and don't leave residue behind.

A sulfate shampoo will be necessary to remove any non-soluble silicone from your hair, so be aware before slathering any on. Silicones that require shampoo to remove include dimethicone and amodimethicone (or any silicone whose name includes "amo," "amine," or "amino"). If silicone isn't removed, it may lead to unhappy hair. The stickier silicones can attract dirt or other gunk, making the hair feel heavy and gross.

If you love what silicones do for your hair, don't feel guilty about using them in moderation—just make sure to pick the right ones for your routine.

MINERAL OIL

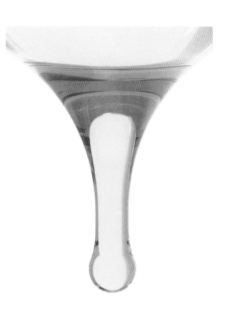

Mineral oil (alternately labeled as paraffin, petrolatum, prolatum oil, white mineral oil, or petroleum) is sometimes added to hair products to condition and protect hair and minimize static. You may have read some posts on no-poo forums claiming that mineral oil is added to beauty products because, as a petroleum byproduct, its ubiquity makes it cheaper to add to things than to dispose of. I can't find any solid evidence that this is actually true.

If it were true, would mineral oil be a problematic ingredient? There's some suggestion among health and beauty bloggers that mineral oil interferes with skin's moisture levels or vitamin absorption or synthesis, but again I could not find a credible source supporting that theory. The reliable information available on mineral oil says that it poses low if any hazard. It may exacerbate acne for some sensitive folks, so abstain if that's the case for you. Otherwise, it seems fine with moderate use.

SODIUM CHLORIDE

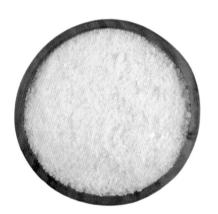

Some hair products contain sodium chloride, aka straight-up salt. Don't worry too much about this one. Its only potential issue is that is may cause dry or irritated skin or interfere with the effectiveness of keratin treatments.

That wraps up our step-by-step survey of what's in a shampoo bottle.

The Takeaway

To summarize our discussion of the general health risks of shampoo, we'll return to the Environmental Working Group. A broad EWG survey comparing over forty thousand products noted that standard shampoos tend to have at least one red-flag ingredient. Of most concern to the EWG are fragrances, parabens, 1,4-dioxane, and DMDM hydantoin. It may be that the levels of these chemicals contained in our cosmetics are low enough not to cause any problem, but if all products use them, then the toxic exposure can accumulate, and can be especially problematic for the tiniest people among us (and as we've seen, baby products are not always free from these contaminants).

Perhaps the biggest issue is the lack of regulations. We aren't told what's in a fragrance, for example. Indeed, cosmetic products *are not regulated* by the FDA (it's not called the Makeup and Shampoo Administration, right?) or any governmental agency. In other words, there is no governmental requirement to test cosmetic products for safety before selling them to the public.

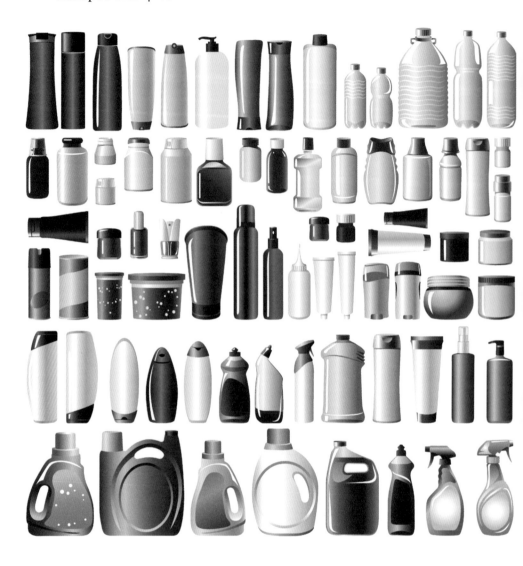

The Environmental Working Group, a non-partisan, non-profit organization, aims to work against that gap through independent research, but the truth is that we simply lack information about how bad—*if* bad—a lot of these chemicals are. According to Jane Houlihan, the EWG's VP of Research, "it's high time for Congress to update standards for cosmetics, and require that companies prove their products are safe for children before they go on store shelves." Hear, hear.

In the meantime, what's a conscientious consumer to do? I'll reiterate that a lot of what the EWG contends *may* be harmful *may* not be. The warnings they give are not meant as guarantees of impending doom—just as analyses of potential risks, big and small, or highlights of what still remains unstudied and hence unknown. In many instances, there's just not enough research to make a truly informed decision. In cases like this, I like to do my own analysis: Are the potential risks (big or small) worth the benefit? For something like sunscreen, if my only option is an easy-to-accidentally-inhale-when-standing-downwind spray-on sunscreen bottle filled with the estrogen-mimicking UV blocker oxybenzone (spray-bottle screens and oxybenzone are both no-no's per the EWG's handy sunscreen guide, by the way, which you can find on their website), that's still better than being exposed to the sun without protection, which demonstrably causes cancer big-time, not to mention wrinkles.

The bottom line? When purchasing (or making!) products, use your judgment, and base that judgment on the best facts available.

DIRTY WORDS

If these are on the label of your hair-care product, consider putting it back on the shelf and going with one of the alternatives discussed in this book: sulfates, parabens, phthalates, PEG compounds, anything containing "xynol," "ceteareth," or "oleth," fragrance, triclosan.

TECH TIP

Trying to keep track of all these ingredients can feel like a full-time job. Luckily, smart robots exist to help us be less burdened by information overload. Check out the Think Dirty app. It allows you to scan a product with your smartphone to get all the dirty details on what's inside.

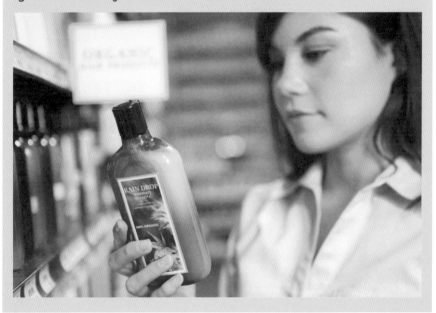

Worth It?

Apart from the potential risks, how useful are shampoo ingredients?

In other words, are they so stupendous at their job that they are worth any possible problems? The short answer is no. Sodium lauryl sulfate and the like are very effective detergents, but your hair is not

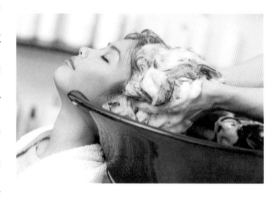

a set of dirty dishes after a dinner party. Even though shampoo contains much less SLS (shampoo is only about 15 percent SLS; dish detergent is much higher), an even milder cleanser can get the job done as effectively without the potential problems of SLS.

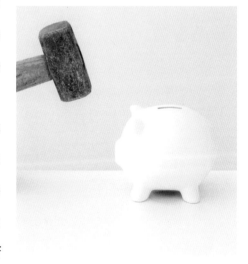

And certain shampoo ingredients are straight-up unnecessary. Do you really need your shampoo to have a pearly appearance? Is that worth paying for? That's the purpose of glycol distearate and other "opacifiers." Even suds, though they may *feel* cleansing, are actually expendable.

Just as advertisers created the myth that daily shampooing is the way to keep us fresh and beautiful as a way to convince us to part with our hard-earned cash, the shampoo industry profits from our dependence on that daily dose of sudsy, pearly, fragrant detergent. But we can profit from avoiding it. You don't need to buy what they're selling to have great hair. The shampoo-free lifestyle carries the added benefit of being (for the most part) crazy cheap!

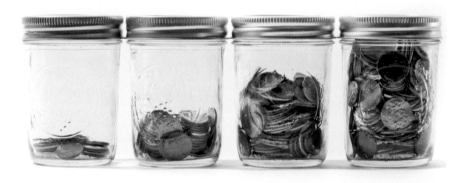

A box of baking soda and a bottle of apple cider vinegar will cost less than a cheap drugstore shampoo and last far longer. A 32-ounce bottle of Dr. Bronner's castile soap costs around $16, but it can last you for *years*. Lots of folks who've permanently shelved shampoo have done it for the savings alone.

Don't forget that big-brand shampoos are diluted with water so you have to use more of them and hence buy them more often. One

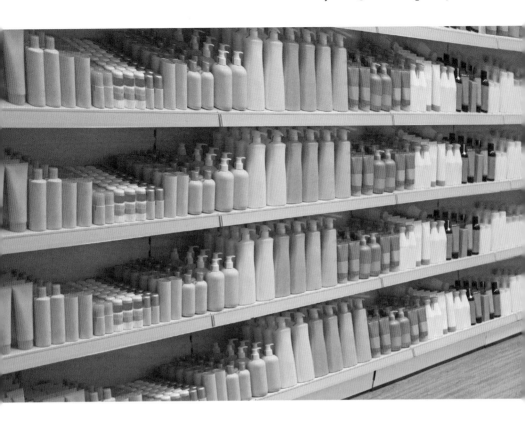

marketing firm estimates that a total of over $4 billion dollars is spent on shampoo and conditioner in a year. Yes, billion with a *B*, and one year: singular. That's a lot of cash washed down the drain.

If you are lucky enough to have cash to burn and would rather invest it in your hair care than actually burn it, consider shelling out for a high-quality product made with you and the planet in mind. You often get what you pay for when it comes to store-bought beauty products. There are some really nice "low poo" (sulfate-, paraben-, general-gunk-free) products on the market, which we'll discuss in greater detail later.

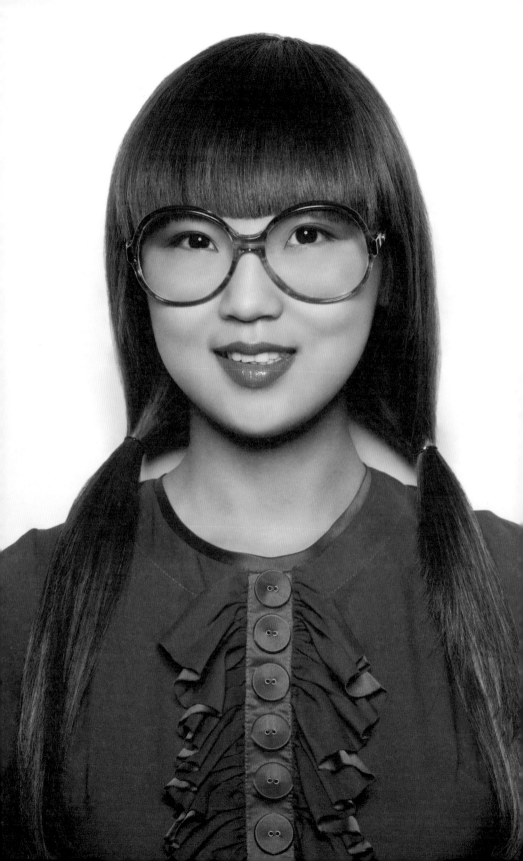

Po(o)llution

One final environmental consideration is the bottle itself. Plastic is a problem not so much because plastic itself is so awful, but more because there's so freaking much of it. Since plastic production began in the 1950s, we've gone from making around 1.5 millions tons of it each year to making 250 million tons. So much of our plastic is 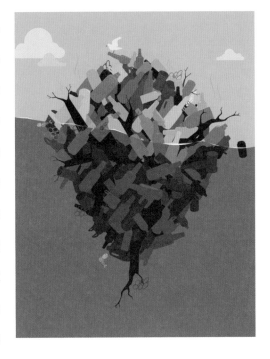 "use it, then lose it." Just think of how many plastic water bottles, takeout containers, Ziploc bags, and other containers you use once and then discard. It's daunting—hard for our little brains to comprehend—and a lot of it is ending up in landfills or in places it shouldn't be, like our oceans.

Plastic biodegrades so slowly that the first plastic to find its way to the ocean is probably still hanging out there. And much of the plastic, rather than biodegrading, just breaks into smaller and smaller pieces, making cleanup close to impossible and wreaking unknown havoc on the marine ecosystem. Look up the "Great Pacific Garbage Patch" if you want to be further depressed about the enormous oceanic trash vortexes plastic pollution has resulted in. It's not known exactly how much plastic reaches the ocean each year, but the figure is well into the millions of tons.

So how does your personal use of shampoo contribute to this? If you use one ounce of shampoo each day, and your typical bottle is about fifteen ounces, that's about twenty-five bottles a year—fifty bottles if you're conditioning too. If you count up all the years you've been shampooing, you could fill a few bathtubs with all that waste.

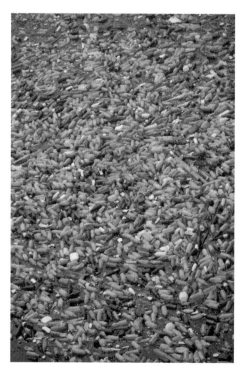

Want to think on a bigger scale? About 1 million pounds of shampoo bottles (only shampoo!) are thrown away by New York City residents every year. Or how about this: If only ⅟₇ of the world's population used only one bottle of shampoo per year, that still makes 1 *billion* plastic shampoo bottles per year! Double that if you count conditioner as well. Even if you recycle, plastic recycling requires energy and has limitations—it's not as earth-friendly as never using the plastic bottle in the first place.

Any way to reduce one's plastic footprint will prove enormously helpful to the planet. Most of the techniques for going shampoo-free will result in a significant decrease in the amount of plastic waste your hair-care routine produces. So help a planet out.

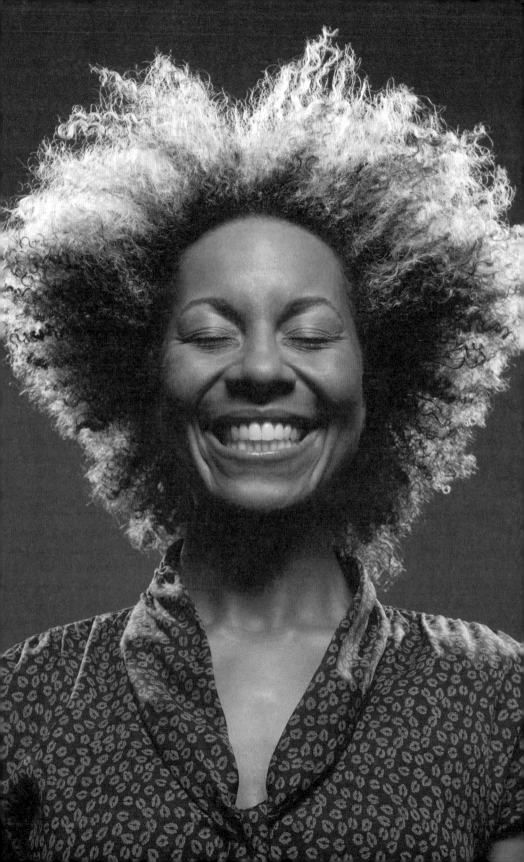

Mirror, Mirror

Okay, we've tackled the health aspects, the financial aspects, the environmental concerns, but what about the most important factor of all (kidding!—mostly . . .): vanity! Can you still be the fairest of them all without shampoo? Most people who quit shampoo for good say that the look and feel of 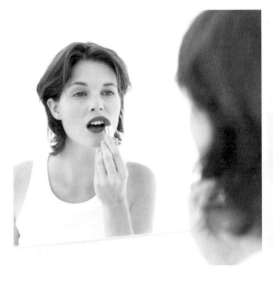 their hair improves. They report hair that's softer, shinier, wavier, and all around better. If that's not true of your hair after you've been with your shampoo-free routine for a while, it's probably time to switch up your technique (it doesn't mean it's time for a shampoo relapse).

The benefits to a shampoo-free lifestyle don't always stop at hair. Many adherents report less acne. They find that their skin was reacting to the shampoo and that once they stop using it, their oil production regulates and their acne clears up. Sodium

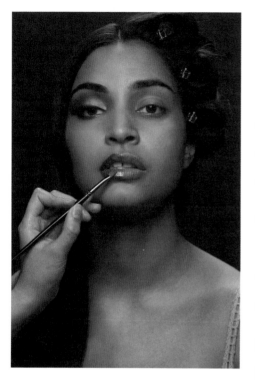

lauryl sulfate messing with your sebum production can have a huge impact on oil production around your hair zone. If you get crazy acne and aren't sure why, especially if you break out around your hairline or where hair touches your body, shampoo may have something to do with it. Conditioner may also be a problem. If it's not detergent, then silicone, panthenol (a form of vitamin B), or petroleum could be the culprit behind hair care–related acne. Quitting the shampoo-then-soften routine may help clear up your skin.

Some guys I've talked to report that going poo-free has substantially slowed their hair loss, and some hair specialists do agree that the detergents, thickeners, alcohols, fragrances, and mineral oils in shampoo may cause hair damage that the body is less able to cope with over time, thus accelerating hair loss. It may be worth quitting shampoo if you're thinning and you'd rather not be.

Of course, many of the "mights" and "maybes" on the benefits of quitting shampoo are based on anecdotal evidence. I wish there was more actual research examining how different hair-care routines affect us, but at the moment, there's not. (Scientists and future scientists, take note!) Just because some people think a certain practice is having a certain effect on them a) doesn't mean it truly is and b) doesn't mean it'll have that effect on you. That said, weigh the benefits on your own by evaluating your own experiences.

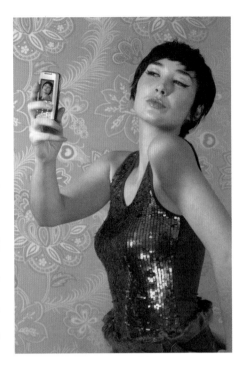

Whether forgoing shampoo will magically cure your acne or halt your hair loss remains to be seen; there's no proof it will (or won't). Regardless, there are other compelling reasons to reevaluate your use of shampoo: from the fact that advertisers and shampoo companies are the ones who convinced us we needed it, to the fact that many of the common shampoo ingredients can have adverse effects on our health and environment, to the sake of your cash-strapped wallet. Whatever your reasons, read on to learn how to take the next step.

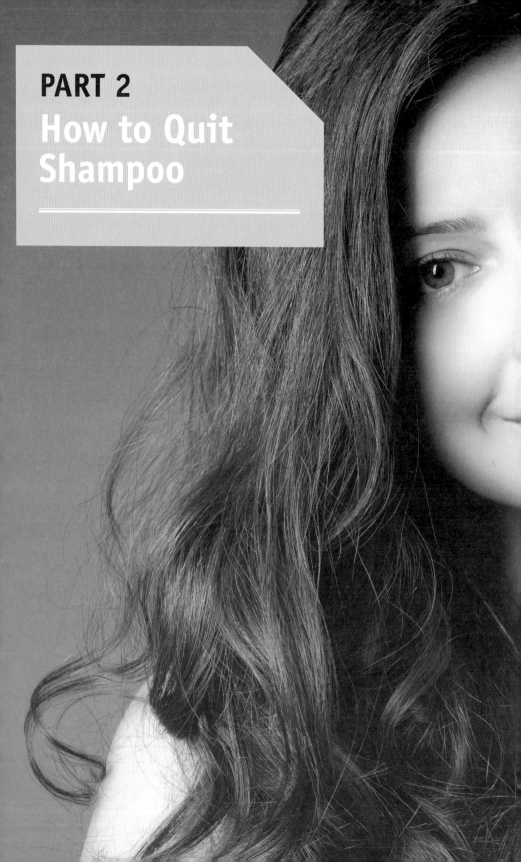

PART 2
How to Quit Shampoo

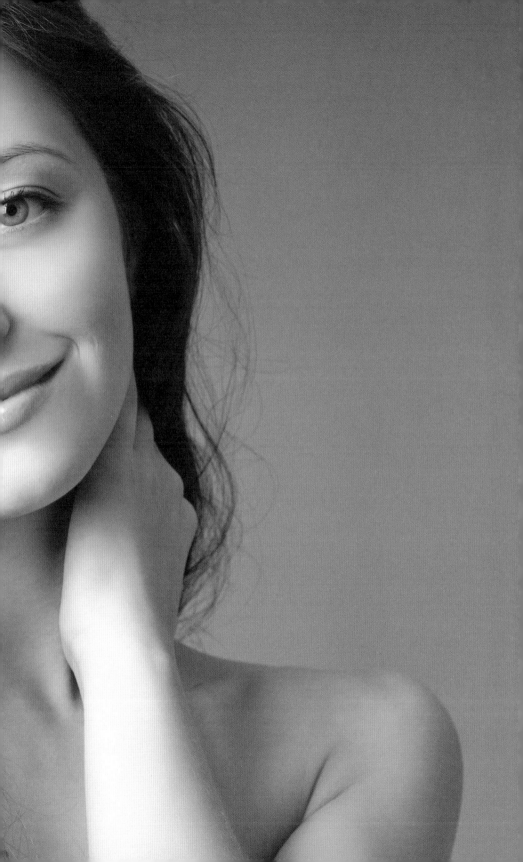

We've tackled the many reasons to leave shampoo behind, and if you found them compelling enough to inspire your own journey to freedom, now you need the details. Just how does one go about permanently setting sham and poo aside? It helps to understand first precisely what shampoo does— what we want it to do and what we don't necessarily need it to do. We've already covered some of this in our discussion of common shampoo ingredients, but let's take a closer look at the process itself. Then, we'll explore all the methods you can use to replicate that process, sans shampoo.

How Shampoo Works

Now that we have a handle on what basic ingredients shampoo entails, it's time for a mini science lesson on how they all function together. To start, let's look at plain soap. What is it, exactly?

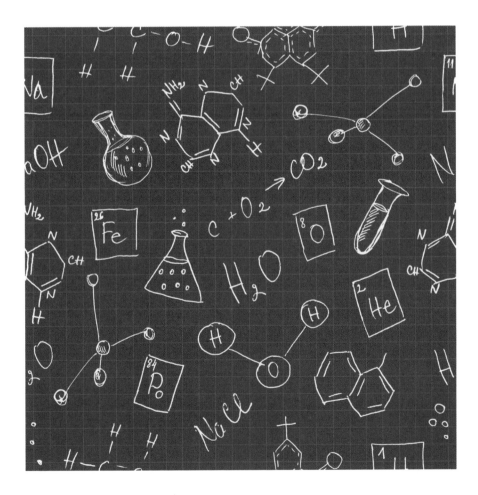

Put simply, soap is a chemical reaction between an acid and an alkali (or "base"). An oil or fat is typically the acid; the alkali historically was ash but later became sodium hydroxide (or potassium hydroxide for liquid soaps), which means that soap is actually a type of salt. You may see ingredients in certain soaps that are "saponified," such as the "saponified coconut oil" in Dr. Bronner's castile soaps. Saponification refers to the process of making a fat into soap by adding an alkali. The word is often said

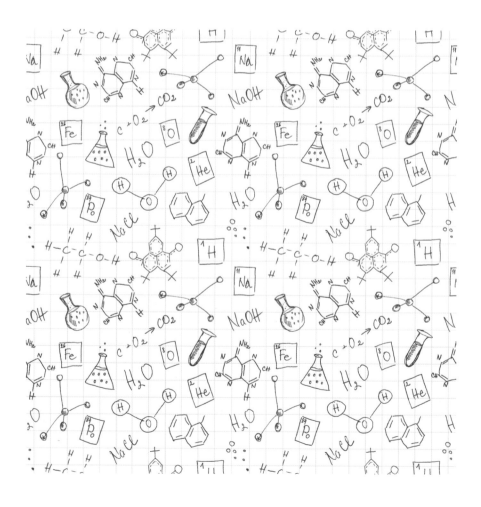

to owe its origin to Sapo Hill, a mythic mountain where ancient Romans sacrificed animals. The story goes that the stream below the mountain became a popular place to wash clothing—it seemed to make them cleaner. Then it was discovered that when the fat drippings from the sacrifices combined with ash from the sacrificial fires, the runoff mixing into the water produced a natural soap. The tale is probably apocryphal, but it does get the basic science right. In actuality, the word soap probably comes from the Gaulish *sapo* or the Germanic *saipa*—both of which correlate to the Latin *sebum* (sound familiar?), which means "fat."

Moving on in time, for all its magical cleaning power, soap has had its drawbacks, like the fact that it leaves scummy residue when used in hard water. Enter detergents. These are chemically

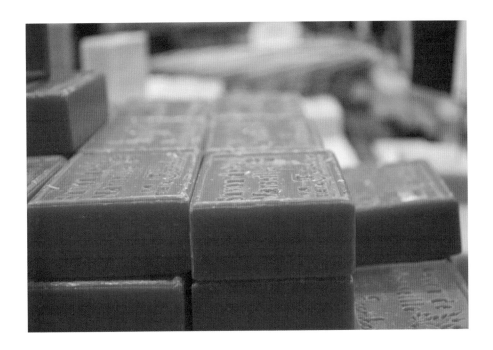

composed soap-like substances that will bind to dirt and grease, but work when soap might not, like in cold water, hard water, or saltwater. Detergents contain surfactants (like our old friend SLS), fatty acid compounds that attach to the gunk on surfaces to allow it to be rinsed away.

This is how shampoo works. It's a mixture of detergents and other materials (softeners, preservatives, and so on) that works to trap the dirt and grease in our hair within a molecular structure that is then rinsed away by water.

What oil is this shampoo attempting to remove? That would be sebum, our skin and scalp's natural oil secretions. Sebum's job (one of them) is to protect our hair, specifically to keep the protein structure from breaking, and it does that job very well. But it also tends to get gunky, trapping skin, dirt, and grease; that's what's happening when our hair gets dirty. The job we want our shampoo to do is remove the grime that attaches to excess scalp oil as well as any dead skin cells. Shampoos made with surfactants will indeed do this, yet still leave the hair relatively soft feeling, which is why they are so popular. Yet when a surfactant shampoo strips away the dirt, grease, and oil, it essentially does its job too well. These detergents are so effective that, when they are used as shampoos, they can strip too much oil, creating the need for conditioner.

Without adequate sebum protection, our hair's protein structure is at risk of damage. It also possible that when the scalp is left bare and insufficiently conditioned, the oil glands then rush to restore the balance, resulting in grease we don't need, and hastening our next shampoo rendezvous.

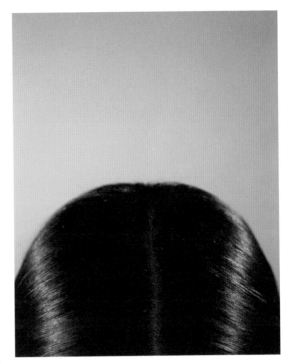

So how can we get the benefits of shampoo without the drawbacks? A nice range of methods can help you accomplish the good that shampoo does, without the accompanying muck (our old friends sham and poo).

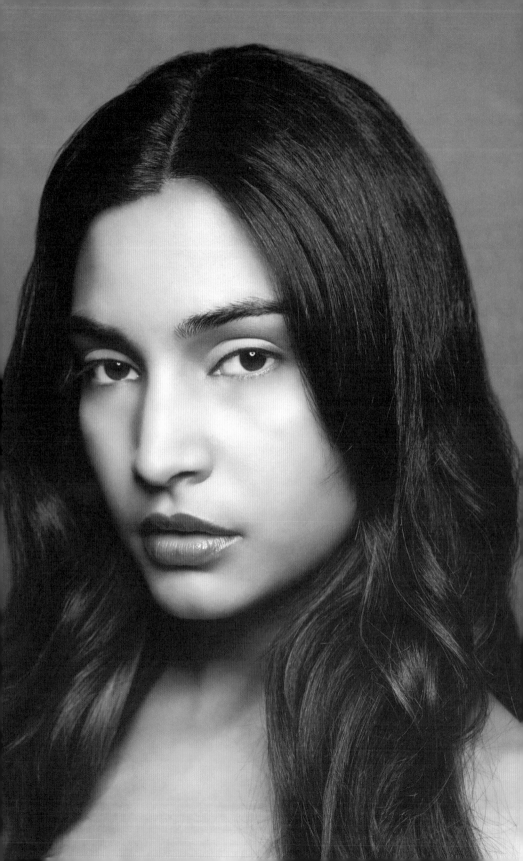

Set Yourself Free

Brass tacks time. There are a few substitutes for the traditional shampoo + condition routine. This section will detail them all, and help you select which method(s) might work best for your hair.

First, an overview of the main options: To replace shampoo, you can try baking soda, castile soap, another type of alkaline wash, soap nuts, conditioner only, bentonite clay or other types of mud washes, aloe vera, or dry shampoo. For a conditioner alternative, you can use acidic options like apple cider vinegar, citrus juice, coffee, or tea, and/or conditioning options like beer, aloe vera, or plant-based oils. Cassia and other herb powders, raw honey, eggs, and a handful of other ingredients can provide benefits of both traditional

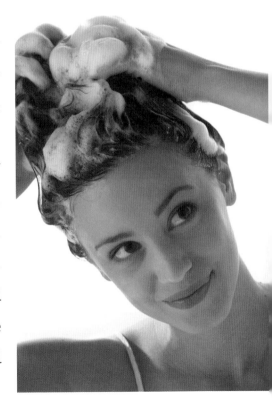

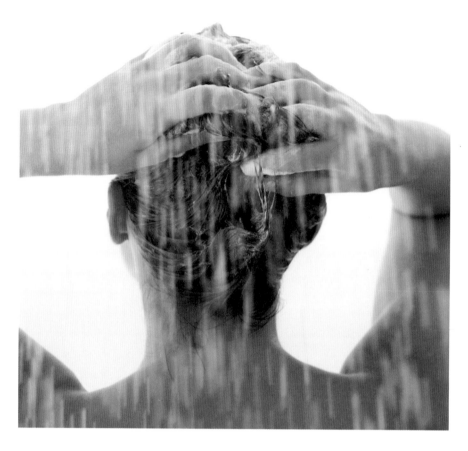

shampoos *and* conditioners. If you're really lucky, simply showering (with water alone) might do the trick.

Obviously, it's not just a matter of throwing all these options on your head and hoping for the best. Your head is not a salad bar. Let's talk methodology, one option at a time.

Step 1: Clean

Are you ready for some cringe-worthy pH puns? Let's start with the *basics*. The standard no-poo routine involves a basic (alkaline) wash, an acidic rinse, and an optional moisturizer. There are a handful of options for your alkaline wash.

BAKING SODA

When people say they are "no poo," this is often what they mean. Baking soda is a commonly touted alternative to shammy poo. It's pretty simple to use: Just mix baking soda with water, apply to the head, massage around your scalp, and rinse.

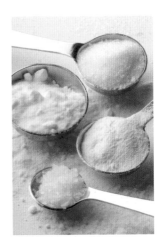

Baking soda is great for a whole range of cleansing activities (just like SLS!). A good starting point for use as a hair cleanser is to mix a half-teaspoon of baking soda with a cup of water. Move up or down from there (the recommended maximum is about one tablespoon per cup) as you figure out how to achieve your best results.

Be careful not to use too much baking soda—less is more, so take it slow. If you have long hair, start with one teaspoon

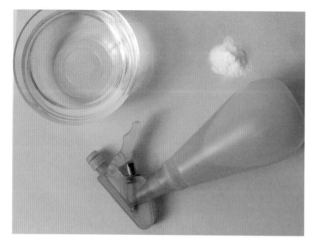

of baking soda and two cups of water. It may be helpful to mix these together and then pour them into an empty shampoo or spray bottle to make the mixture easier to administer. You won't experience lather with a baking soda wash; instead what you're aiming for is a nice feeling of slickness—that should mean you've got the measurements right. You don't want gritty liquid in the bottle, although you can make a baking soda paste to rub into your scalp if that's easier than mixing with warm water for your wash—that may be a better option for those with short hair. Rinse it out right away or leave it on for up to a minute (experiment to see what works best for you). If your hair feels brittle or dry afterward, cut (back on) the BS (ha ha).

Note that it's important to do an acidic rinse after a baking soda wash to return the pH of your hair back closer to neutral. It's also best to keep the baking soda action concentrated to your roots rather than the length of your hair. If you're using a baking soda wash and acid rinse, you'll also probably want to intermittently use a "carrier oil" for conditioning. Carrier oils (different from essential oils) are oils derived from plant fats (coconut, olive, etc.) used to moisturize. They are called carrier oils because essential oils or other extracts can be safely added to them for use.

CASTILE SOAP

Castile soap is easy to use, and it even produces some lather, for a sudsy feeling that you'll enjoy if you're fond of that sensory element of shampooing. Try a strongly diluted version first (you can always add more soap to the mix if it's not getting the job done) because some people find castile soap's cleansing action to be too strong when undiluted. Be aware, though, that if you dilute

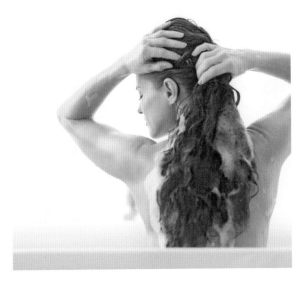

the mixture ahead of time, any preservative ingredients won't work as well, so don't leave the diluted mixtures sitting in your shower for weeks. A good option is to keep an undiluted mixture in the shower and an empty bottle to dilute it with right before pouring on your head.

Dr. Bronner's is a popular pre-made castile soap. Take a look at the ingredients: pretty simple stuff. Also, enjoy finding the list of

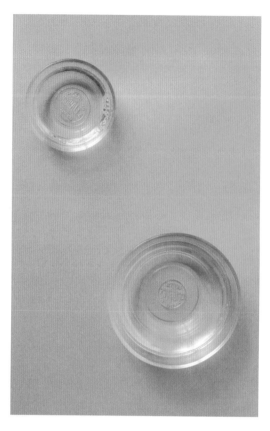

ingredients, because the packaging is filled with tiny-font text—most of it eyebrow-raising, yet somehow aesthetically compelling? It is certain to make shower time more entertaining. (You do you, Dr. B.) The lavender version is a common selection for use on hair.

You can also buy an unscented castile soap and add your own essential oils. Or, make your own castile soap if you're feeling ambitiously DIY. Always follow castile soap with an acid rinse. Use apple cider vinegar, or another acidic option. Dr. B's actually makes a nice citrus rinse specially formulated to follow their castile soap used as shampoo.

A NOTE ON ESSENTIAL OILS

Essential oils can make a nice addition to your shampoo-free routine. Tea tree and lavender are popular for cleansing, jojoba can help protect and add moisture (Dr. Bronner's castile soap

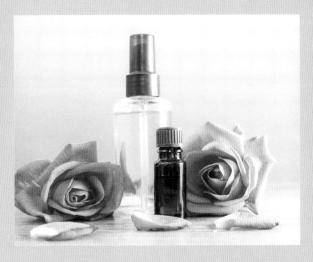

actually contains jojoba already, and they make tea tree and lavender versions), and some oils are worth it for the lovely smell alone.

It's fun to experiment, though be forewarned that essential oils can be pricey. That said, one bottle goes a long way; a drop or two per mixture bottle will be enough. Don't overdo it! You can always add more, but you can't take out oil you've mixed in, so go sparingly until you get your ideal ratio.

Know that essential oils are strong distilled mixtures and many have medicinal properties. Drinking them could mean a call to poison control, to give you an idea of their strength. Different oils have different properties (and different potential hazards). Make sure you are using them safely by checking the Material Safety Data Sheet (these will be available from any good essential

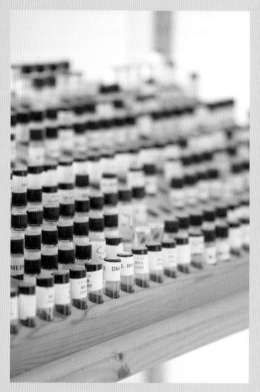

oil manufacturer—if a sheet is not available, probably better not to buy from that company). The sheet will list any risks, ranging from things like "flammable" to "harmful if swallowed" to "dangerous to the ozone layer." Mountain Rose Herbs provides data sheets if you call or write to them.

Essential oils are derived from bark, leaves, or stems of plants, whereas carrier oils are derived from the fatty portions (seeds, nuts, etc.)

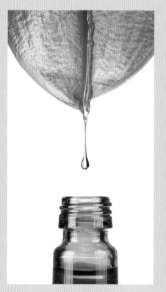

A note on keeping things fresh: Essential oils can evaporate over time if exposed to air. Carrier oils won't evaporate but they will spoil after prolonged oxidation. Best to keep a lid on both. Essential oils can be added to your "soap," your vinegar rinse, or with a carrier oil used as conditioner.

SAPONACEOUS HERBS

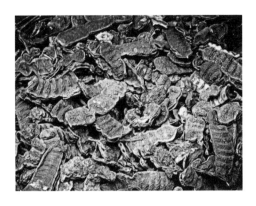

A special set of saponaceous (i.e., "soapy") herbs also make great shampoo substitutes. Shikakai and aritha (also called "reetha" or simply "soap nuts") are two of the most popular. They're fun because being saponified means they'll create that sudsy lather you'll lack if you switch to baking soda. They also impart body and manageability to the hair and may help with dandruff.

When using powdered shikakai or aritha, use the same measurement and method as for baking soda to start out. Ready-to-use versions are also available in soap-bar form or as a liquid mixture. Dr. Bronner's makes a shikakai soap blend if you like the sound of a premixed option (it's another one to follow with a vinegar or acidic rinse). Soap nuts are sometimes

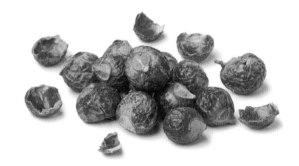

used to treat lice—here's hoping you'll never need them to. You'll also often hear that soap nuts prevent or treat hair loss, but that

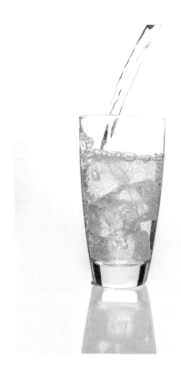

appears to be an untested claim. Go easy on the saponaceous herb use if your hair tends to have dryness issues.

TONIC WATER

Tonic water is basic (in several senses) and thus works as an alkaline cleanser. You could also dissolve Tums in water and use that mixture to the same effect. Either of these methods could be a solution if you find yourself on the road and don't have many options available short notice.

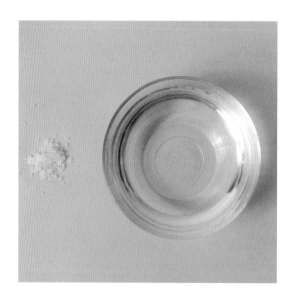

SALT

Salt is another choice if you find yourself without your usual products on hand and are looking to get your hair clean without resorting to a detergent shampoo. Like baking soda, salt is alkaline. Use a pinch when you're in a pinch: Mix with warm water and follow with an acid rinse. A dash of salt can also be added to castile soap to help cut oil and to exfoliate the scalp. Just keep the quantities small—your hair won't be any happier oversalted than your food would be.

Beyond the "basics," a few other options can provide the cleansing action you need without the shampoo you don't.

ALOE VERA

If the traditional basic + acidic method is giving you grief, pH could be to blame. The rapid change from the high pH of an alkaline wash to the low pH of 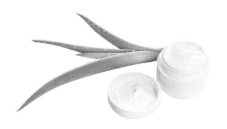 an acidic rinse may not be best for everyone's scalp. Aloe vera has a neutral pH so it's a balanced option—and it works to smooth and moisturize hair. It can soothe a dry scalp and help combat flaking.

Mix aloe vera with glycerin or coconut milk for added cleansing power. It's best to buy pure aloe vera so you're not dealing with any additives that might muck up your hair. Of course, the purest option of all is to take a leaf from your own homegrown aloe plant. Add a few drops of a moisturizing oil to the mix, and you just may be able to skip an added conditioner. Easy and good for you!

CO-WASHING

This method is particularly good if you have curly hair. It's a popular non-poo method among those with tight curls, in the 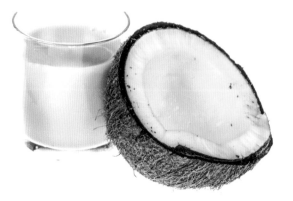 3A to 4C range of hair types, but it can work wonders on looser waves as well. Shampoo can be exceptionally harsh on curly hair because much of the scalp's natural oil tends to stay close to the scalp and may not make it all the way down the length of the hair, making shampoo extra stripping. Conditioner has cleansing agents in it that are much milder

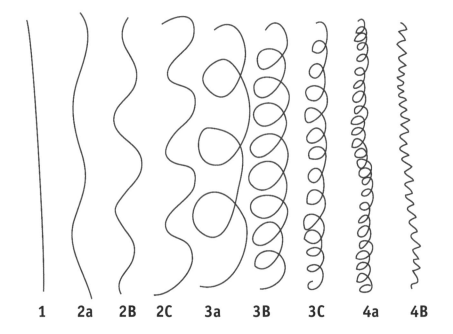

| 1 | 2a | 2B | 2C | 3a | 3B | 3C | 4a | 4B |

than the sulfates in shampoo.

Co-washing means washing your hair with conditioner—and conditioner only. Some co-washers will do a shampoo wash every few weeks, while others avoid shampoo entirely and use baking soda, clay washes, a low-poo option, or another shampoo alternative. When selecting a brand, read

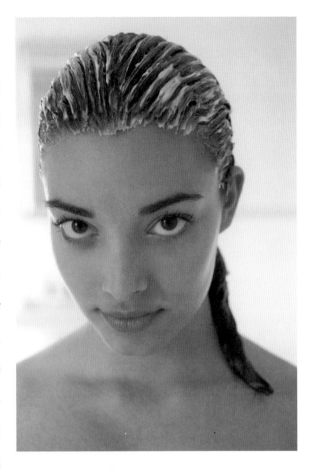

the ingredients and watch out for the dirty words we talked about earlier. NEUMA and SheaMoisture offer safe bets.

Co-washing can also be a good solution if you're caught in a pinch, say when traveling or staying outside your home, and you don't want to resort to shampoo.

GET PLOPPY

If you have naturally curly hair, you may also wish to look into plopping: a method for getting your curls looking their best without blow-drying or other heat. It involves "plopping" your hair down onto a cloth (not a towel, as a towel will prove too thick

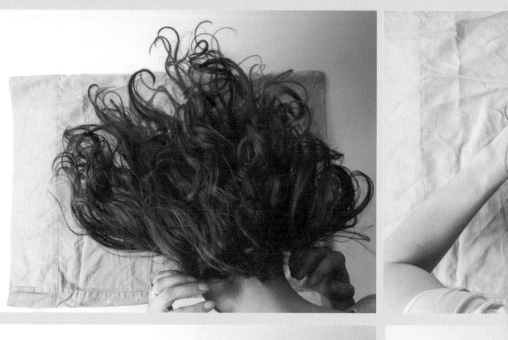

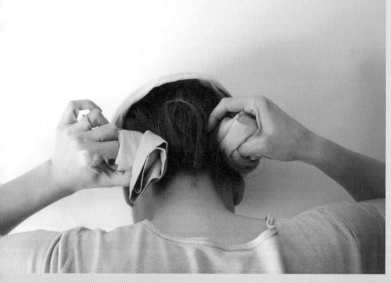

and absorbent), which you then tie or secure around your head so that your curls are stacked on top of your head as they dry. Use a pillowcase or an old T-shirt. Watch some tutorial videos online to see a live-action demonstration and you'll get the hang of it in no time.

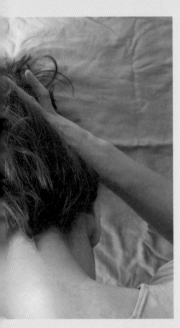
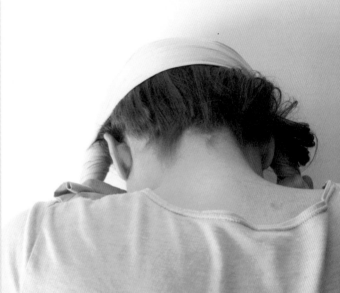
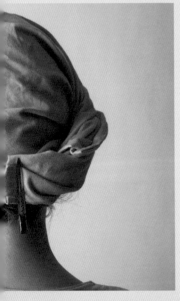
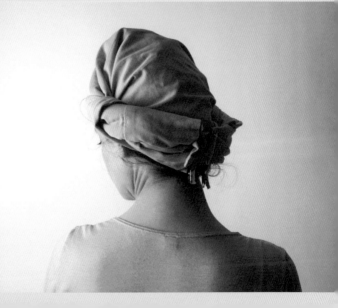

CLAYS AND MUDS

Picture people relaxing in a spa with clay smeared all over their face. Do they just love having dirt spread all over their pores? Or what's the secret? Turns out clay or mud masks are actually good

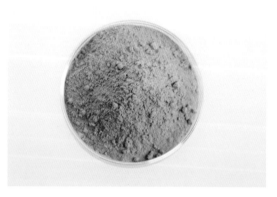

at absorbing impurities—meaning they make good cleansers. Clay can be used similarly for hair. Ideally, it will draw out the gunk and grime without messing too much with the natural oils, which makes it popular among curly-haired folks.

Clay tends to leave curls soft and with a nice shape, and it provides the hair nutrients and shine. Less is more for this one; if you use too much, it'll dry your hair right out. Clay can be fun because it will affect the texture of your hair, making it more moldable, as though it had product in it. Similar to baking soda, try about a teaspoon of clay to a cup of warm water at first and see where that leaves you. If your hair dries out, you're using too much. Avoid mixing the clay in a metal bowl.

Look for bentonite, kaolinite, or rhassoul clay and be sure to get the good stuff: The powder should be gray or cream; white means it's probably not the best quality. Bentonite clay typically comes from volcanic ash. Most bentonite clay available for purchase was mined from deposits in Wyoming and Montana. Other types of clay like kaolinite are coal-related. Rhassoul clay is another nice option. It comes from a Moroccan mountain range and has been used in Moroccan hair-care traditions for hundreds of years. Some fans of clay enjoy mixing the clay powder with apple

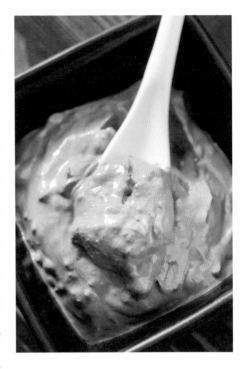

cider vinegar, aloe vera juice, coconut milk, and/or essential and carrier oils. You want the mixture you apply to your head to have the consistency of yogurt (no matter what ingredients are in it). Look online for recipes or experiment.

HONEY

Using honey on your hair has a few perks. Honey is a humectant, meaning that it helps your hair lock in moisture. If your hair is dried out—from heat, sun, or your other hair products—honey can help restore it. Honey's also an emollient, so it smoothes and softens as it moisturizes. The benefits don't stop there: Honey is antibacterial, antifungal, and an antioxidant—all good news for your hair and scalp. Honey enthusiasts say it cuts down on frizz and dandruff, while leaving hair soft and improving hair texture.

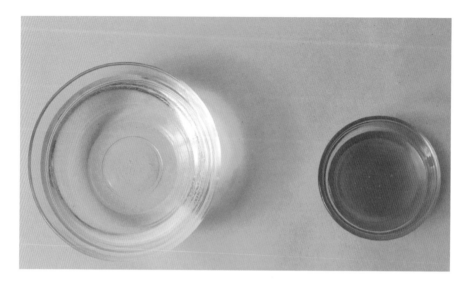

For honey shampoo, use raw honey (to ensure all its kickass properties haven't been pasteurized into oblivion). Mix honey with warm water, at about one part honey to three or four parts water. Add a few drops of your favorite essential oil, if you like. If the honey won't dissolve, heat the mixture until it melts, but keep the temperature low. Massage the mixture into wet hair in the shower, concentrating on the scalp, and rinse. You'll want to make small batches of honey shampoo and use them up quickly—spoilage can occur when the honey is diluted with water. Another tip: Don't overdo it or your hair will become greasy. You may want to alternate honey use with another poo-free method. Some people benefit from a vinegar rinse after honey, but you may not need one.

EGGS

Eggs actually have a lot to offer, hair-care wise. Both the whites and the yolks can be used for different purposes. Egg whites can be separated and mixed into the hair as a shampoo. Because they contain enzymes that eat bacteria, egg whites work well to remove oils. So if, for example, you do a hot oil deep conditioning mask without realizing that you need a shampoo to rinse it out, and baking soda or water just won't cut it, try an egg white mixture to de-grease. Keep in mind that the egg needs to stay raw; mind your water temperature when you rinse so nothing gets scrambled.

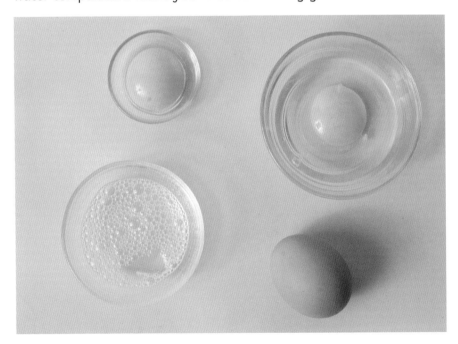

The yolks are useful too. Check out the conditioning section below for more details. You could even try using the whole egg

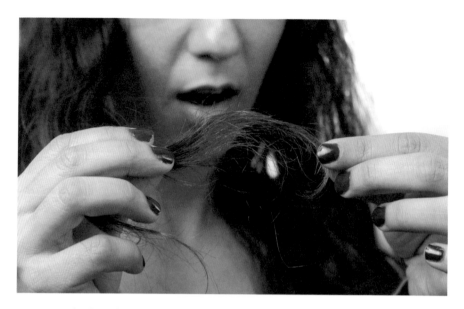

on your hair: the total package. But watch out for egg overuse. Too much protein can cause your hair to split or break. Not a good look. And note that eggs can also strip color out of hair, as well as grease.

DRY "SHAMPOO"

Dry shampoo is really handy if you're seeing grease build up between washes. (It can be a lifesaver during the detox period.) Rather than go with a store-bought aerosol can, it's easy (and healthy and safe) to use a DIY alternative. Make your own with cornstarch, baking soda, or arrowroot. Adding cocoa or cinnamon helps camouflage the shampoo on darker hair (just add enough to get the color you're looking for). Adding a few drops of your favorite essential oil scent will leave you smelling great.

Dry shampoo is a great on-the-go solution. Sprinkle a little on your greasy spots using an old saltshaker or powder container, or use a makeup brush to apply. Comb through your hair to distribute the powder and remove any excess, and voila! If your dark hair shows the powder even with cocoa added (or you don't

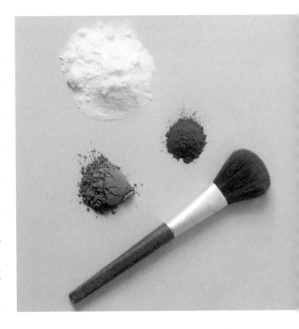

want to add cocoa), applying at night will give your hair time to absorb the powder, meaning less white residue when you leave the house in the morning. Remember, grease isn't the same as dirt, so you may be able to really stretch your washes by supplementing with dry shampoo.

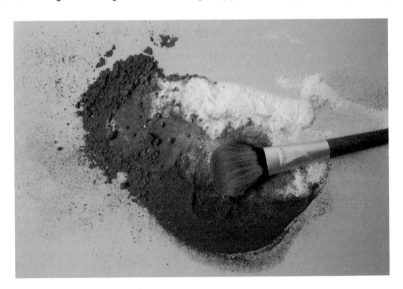

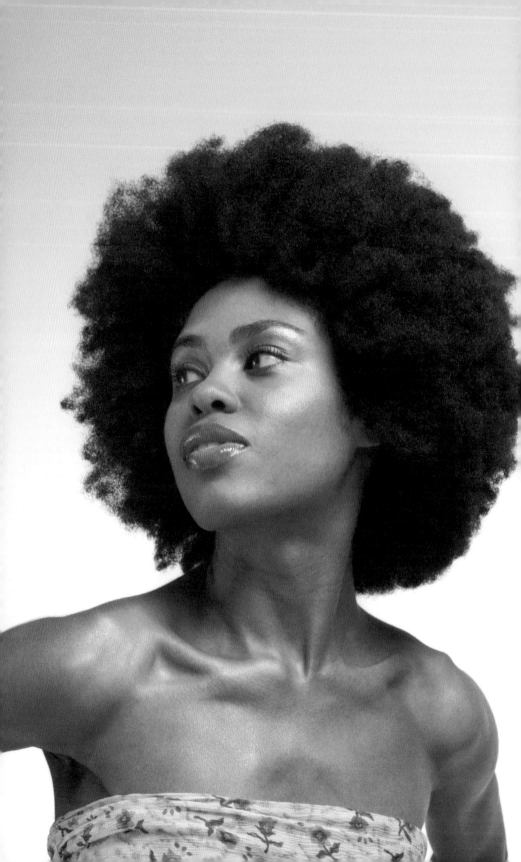

Step 2 (and/or Step 3): The Other Half

What about conditioner? You should no longer need to replace oils stripped out of your hair like you would with traditional shampooing methods, but you will still want to follow up your cleansing with a conditioning treatment of some kind.

There are two elements to this. One is that if you're now using an alkaline cleanser, you will want to use an acidic rinse to manage the pH and help your hair stay soft, manageable, and properly balanced. The other is that even if you're not stripping your hair's oils with sulfates, you may still benefit from added moisture. Let's delve into the different possibilities for these two types of post-cleaning options in more detail.

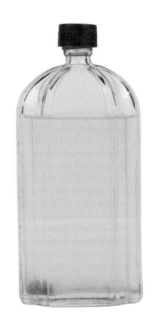

PERFECT YOUR PH

First comes acid. Not the 1960s Haight-Ashbury kind, but the kind that's less than 7 on the pH scale. Using an acidic rinse is more about clarifying your hair than it is conditioning it in the traditional sense. Think of the soap scum that sometimes builds up in our faucets and tubs. A similar residue can be left in your hair if you're using an ingredient like baking soda instead of sodium lauryl sulfate. Acid can help remove any scum—or deposits from hard water.

Acidity will also bring your hair's pH back into balance (closer to neutral) after an alkaline cleansing. If you're using a basic wash, you'll want to follow it with one of the following options.

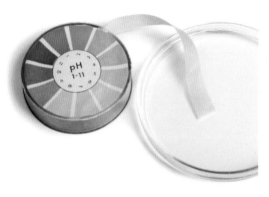

Thoroughly rinse after your basic wash before applying your acid rinse to avoid any unintentional chemistry science fair volcanoes. If you're worried that pH issues may affect your hair health, buy some home testing strips to make sure your mixtures stay within the safe zone (around 5 is probably optimal, and below 4 or above 8 could be problematic).

Apple Cider Vinegar

The most common alternative to conditioner among the no-poo crowd is apple cider vinegar. ACV will remove leftover residue, and its low pH helps assure hair and scalp will be left in the best

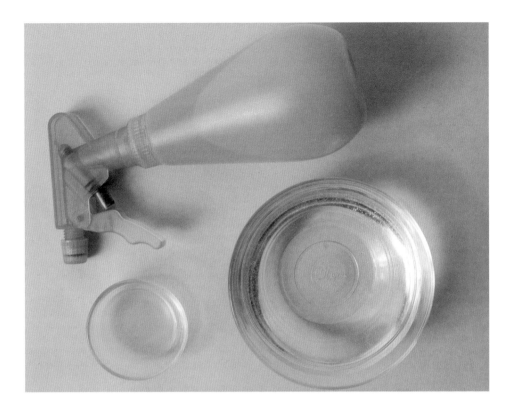

shape after a high-pH wash. For mixture proportions, begin with a strongly diluted version and bump it up a notch as needed (as with alkalis, better to start low on the acid level). One teaspoon to a cup is a good jumping-off point. Premix or mix as you go. A spray bottle makes for easy application. You may want to concentrate more on the length of hair rather than the scalp, but as always, experiment. You can also play around with how long you leave the mixture on your head—some people have better results after letting the ACV marinate for a few minutes. Just be careful your mixture isn't too strong in that case—if the pH is too low, it can damage your hair. Rinse thoroughly to get rid of that briny smell.

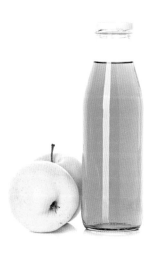

Some vinegar users report having more luck with white vinegar than apple cider, but be extra cautious with white vinegar as it's stronger—dilute, dilute, dilute. Claims of ACV's general magical healing powers abound, but not much research has been done yet to support them.

Citrus Juice

Another acidic option is juice from a lemon or other citrus fruit, such as lime, orange, or grapefruit. If you can't seem to escape the vinegar smell using ACV, experiment with these fruits. Even if you don't have issues with vinegar leaving you less than rosy, why not experiment to see what citrus has to offer?

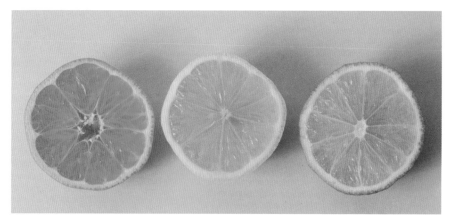

As with any acidic mixture, start out diluted. Try one part citrus juice to two parts water for your first batch. See how it compares to vinegar. Does your scalp like one more than the other? Does your hair look shinier with lemon than with lime? It may be worth trying a few different acidic methods to see what leaves your hair in the best shape. If you're looking to lighten your hair naturally, citrus juice may do the trick. If you're not, use it sparingly.

Citric Acid

You can turn to citric acid (the powdered kind) for your acid rinse as well. It's another good bet if leftover vinegar odor proves difficult to conquer. You can find citric acid in a big grocery store, often near canning supplies. (While you're mastering the art of ditching shampoo, why not start canning too?)

Mix the powder (⅛ of a teaspoon or less should be enough) with warm water and heat to melt it. Return the liquid to a skin-safe temperature before pouring it on your head; use the same rinsing method as for a vinegar rinse, but be careful not to leave it on too long. Some people report success mixing the powder with cool water and shaking to ensure even distribution before applying. Don't accidentally buy ascorbic acid instead of citric acid, and know that overuse can be problematic for hair color and hair health. Keep the dose low, and monitor your hair for signs of unhealthiness.

Coffee and Tea

If you don't finish your morning mug of coffee or tea, put the liquid leftovers to good use. Coffee and tea are acidic and can be used as a post-cleansing rinse. No need to dilute unless you brew your beverages superhumanly strong; after all, coffee and tea are already diluted. Coffee many help to minimize hair shedding, and tea can help leave your hair shiny. Be aware that coffee and tea can affect hair color (with hair becoming more like the color of the liquid over time). This can be a reason to avoid certain brews—or a reason to use them! Leave on a little longer if you're looking to tint, cover gray, or add highlights.

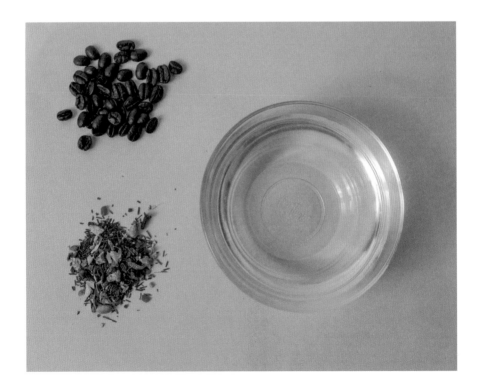

TIP! Whatever your method, stylists swear by a final cool water rinse to help the hair stay frizz-free.

MOISTURIZING AND OTHER "CONDITIONS"

If you were never big on conditioner, you may be fine using just baking soda or castile soap and following with an acidic rinse. But if you are experiencing dry or brittle hair, your hair feels tangled, or your locks are otherwise lacking luster, you'll benefit from a conditioning boost. This could be a once-a-month deep treatment or a lighter moisturizing session after every poo-free wash (similar to traditional conditioner application), or some combination thereof. What can you use to not just remove residue but also condition?

Oils and Butters

There are a few good oil-based options. Coconut oil gets rave reviews, but be careful with this one. It'll leave your hair very soft, but it can't be washed out with just baking soda. Don't do a deep condition

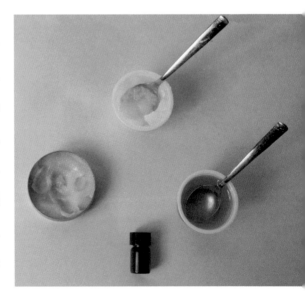

with coconut oil unless you use castile soap or a low-poo option. Some people have also reported success using an egg yolk mixture to remove coconut oil after a deep conditioning treatment. You could give it a shot, but be prepared to use a low-poo solution if the oil won't budge.

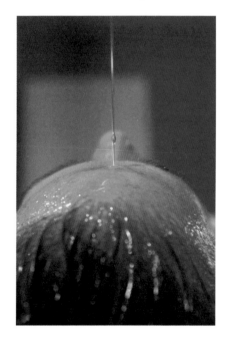

In addition to coconut oil, you can also use olive oil, avocado oil, jojoba oil, sweet almond oil, or the ever-popular argan oil. To boost moisture after a wash, simply place a few drops of your favorite oil on your palm after a shower, rub hands together, then run them down the length of your wet hair (focus on the ends, not the roots). This helps to lock in the moisture. If your hair still feels dry between washings, add a few drops to dry hair using the same method every few days. Aim for even distribution.

To deep condition, use a few tablespoons of oil and massage throughout damp hair, concentrating on the ends. If you have grease issues, skip the scalp, but if you have flakes or dryness, rub oil into the scalp as well. Apply mild heat or wrap a damp warm washcloth around your head. Leave the oil on for as little as twenty minutes and as long as overnight. Try once a month for your deep conditioning treatment.

Shea butter is also a much-loved nut-based hair moisturizer. Curlies in particular should check out its ability to soothe the scalp, seal in moisture along the full length of the hair strand, smooth, soften, and protect from external damage.

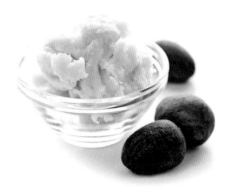

Beer

Beer can be a real boon for your tresses. The wheat, hops, and malt in beer contain proteins, silica, minerals, vitamins, and essential oils that boost hair's body, shine, bounce, and strength—a powerful combination!

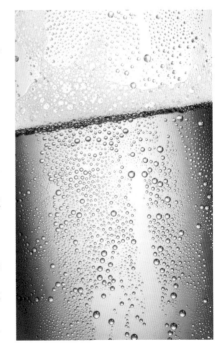

There are several ways to incorporate beer into your beauty routine. You can pour flat beer over wet hair in the shower. Leave for several minutes at least before rinsing with cool water. The alcohol in beer can help cleanse and add shine, but if you have issues with alcohol drying out your hair, reduce the beer over low heat first to remove the alcohol. Let cool before applying. A beer rinse can be applied before or after your non-shampoo cleanser. You can also spritz flat beer onto dry hair as a styling tonic. The smell generally dissipates as the liquid evaporates.

A beer rinse can be done once a month. If you're feeling lazy—or adventurous—Dogfish Head brewery makes a shampoo bar out of their ale, and the BRÖÖ line of hair and skin products (available at Whole Foods) are all beer-based. BRÖÖ's shampoos and conditioners are formulated without most of the bad-guy ingredients discussed earlier. No sulfates, phthalates, or parabens.

Aloe Vera

As we saw in the section on cleansing, aloe can be mixed with other ingredients and used as a shampoo alternative. It can also make for a nice deep-conditioning treatment. Simply massage aloe vera gel thoroughly into damp hair. Put on a shower cap or warm towel, let the aloe do its thing for twenty minutes or so, rinse, and enjoy.

Amla, Tulsi, and More

Amla is a plant-based option for hair conditioning treatments commonly used in traditional Hindu hair care. Fans of amla claim that it moisturizes, strengthens hair, provides texture, fights scalp itch, and reduces hair loss and graying. (Before you spend your hard-earned money, remember these are anecdotal claims, not scientific ones.) Amla comes from the Indian gooseberry and has a potent smell, so be prepared if you decide to give it a go.

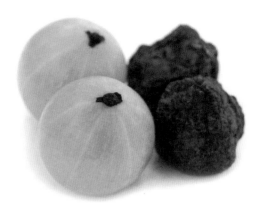

Like amla, tulsi (also known as holy basil) is an Indian plant used in traditional Ayurvedic practice. It is thought to have purifying effects and combat itching, rashes, irritation, and blemishes, which makes it popular for scalp treatment. If you're into Ayurveda, check out bhringraj, brahmi, orange peel, hibiscus, neem, nettle, kalpi tone, and fenugreek (aka methi), all of which are used in Ayurvedic hair treatments. Shikakai and aritha (discussed in the cleaning section) are also Ayurvedic staples, as are cassia and henna, discussed below.

To use amla, tulsi, or any herbal powder, mix the powder with water to create a paste and apply directly to your hair. Wear a shower cap to prevent messy run-off and rinse after fifteen to thirty minutes.

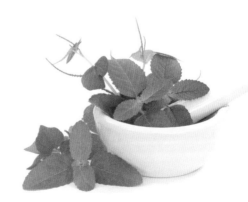

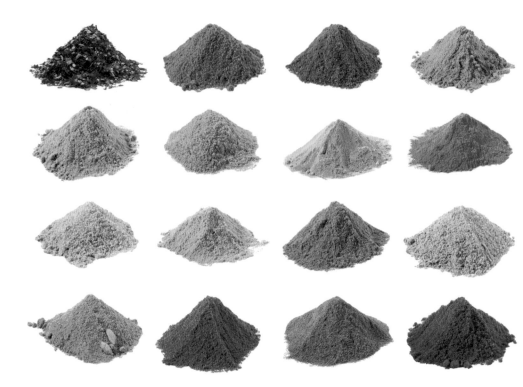

Powdered amla may be a better bet than amla oil, which can be sneakily diluted by manufacturers or contain low levels of amla concentrate.

Henna and Cassia

Henna and cassia are both plant-based powders that can be used to make your hair extra voluminous and silky smooth. They both are also used as natural hair dyes, henna imparting red hues to hair of any shade, and cassia adding a blond tone to light-colored hair. If you don't like the red tinge henna brings, stick to cassia. You'll get the same benefits without the dramatic hue.

Henna and cassia work by coating the hair: smoothing the cuticle and adding strength. Henna is more potent than cassia, so while a cassia treatment will last for a week or two, a henna treatment can last twice as long. (The color of henna is permanent, by the way, though it may fade.) These long-lasting results require some effort up front. To treat your hair with henna,

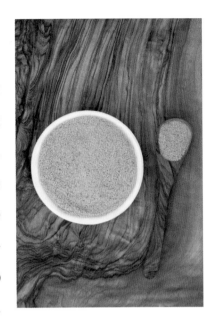

mix the henna powder with water, aiming for yogurt consistency. You'll need to let the mixture sit for a long while (overnight is best). When you apply it to your hair, be very careful, as the mixture can stain anything it touches, including your hands. Wear gloves and consider laying newspaper down over your sink and floor (or wherever you're working with the mix) to catch accidental spills. Put the henna into a plastic bag and cut off the corner for easy application, or use a plastic applicator bottle or a dye

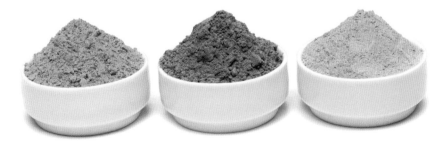

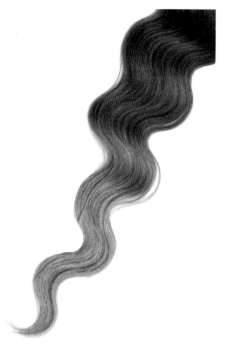

brush (keep in mind, the henna will stain porous plastic). Once you've thoroughly applied, put on a plastic cap and wait for another long while: two hours minimum up to overnight, depending on the level of color action you're looking for.

Cassia is simpler. The mixture only needs thirty minutes to marinate. You don't have to worry about it staining your hands (no gloves needed) or bathroom fixtures. And it doesn't take hours to set. A half hour of letting the mixture saturate your strands should produce optimal results.

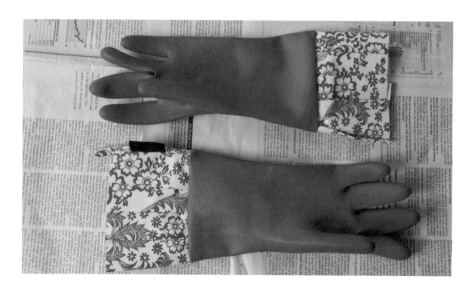

Henna and cassia may affect your curl pattern (making curls looser), particularly immediately after a treatment. Because the effects last so long, it's best to do a strand test before you go for the whole head. Be careful with protein products when using henna. It's best to steer clear of them to avoid breakage. And know that you may need some extra conditioning 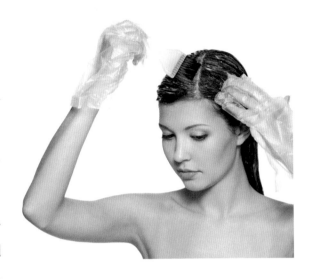 love post-treatment. Make sure the henna and cassia you buy are just that, henna and cassia, and not henna or cassia mixed with other chemicals. Cassia is sometimes called "neutral henna," though it's a different plant entirely.

A few fridge staples provide conditioning power as well. Vegans will want to abstain from any animal-based products, of course.

Yogurt

Thanks to its healthy fats and lactic acid, yogurt makes a nice moisturizer and gentle cleanser. Apply plain yogurt to damp hair (no sugary kinds, and whole milk is best) and let sit for half an hour. Then rinse and follow with your usual cleansing routine.

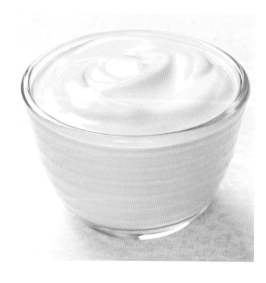

If you like the look of your hair after a yogurt treatment, feel free to add one in every other week.

Egg Yolk

As the albumen (whites) of eggs can be used to clean, the yolk can be used to condition. Yolks can be particularly helpful for long hair that benefits from extra protein. Massage the yolks in, let sit for twenty minutes, and rinse with lukewarm water. Don't do this after every wash. An overdose on protein will damage your hair. Stick to once a month.

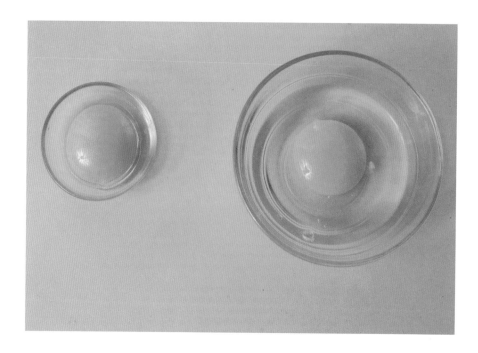

HONEY

Honey is mentioned in the shampoo alternatives section, but it can also be used for a deep conditioning treatment. Mix undiluted raw honey with a little olive oil and massage into your hair and scalp. Apply light heat—a warm washcloth wrapped around the head works great. Or use a shower cap and gentle heat from a blow-dryer. Leave for thirty minutes and then rinse.

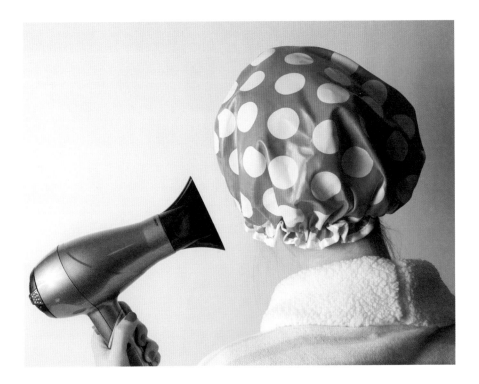

MIX IT UP!

Many of these ingredients can be combined according to your hair's needs and your personal tastes. And your kitchen may already house an abundance of hair-healthy options. Try a whole avocado mashed together with aloe and a spoonful of mayonnaise, honey mixed with vinegar, or coconut milk added to your castile soap. There are tons of options and tons of recipes

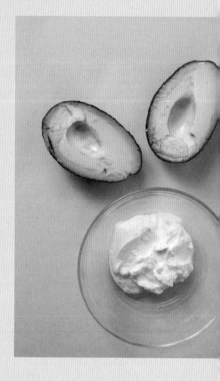

online. Test a few or have fun creating your own concoctions.

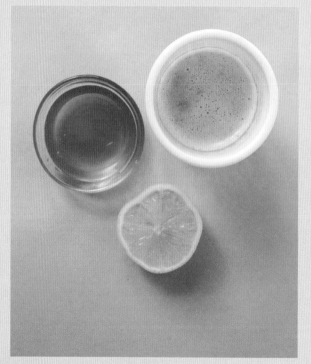

H$_2$O On Its Own

There's one final poo-free method to look at, before we move on to the "low-poo" options. Known on no-poo message boards as the ROM (rinse only method), this is the holy grail of shampoo freedom. In theory, pure water has a pH very close to neutral (Chemistry 101: Less than 7 is acidic; higher than 7 is basic.) But in practice, the pH level of water varies widely by location. Using water only to wash your hair sounds like a dream come true, but be

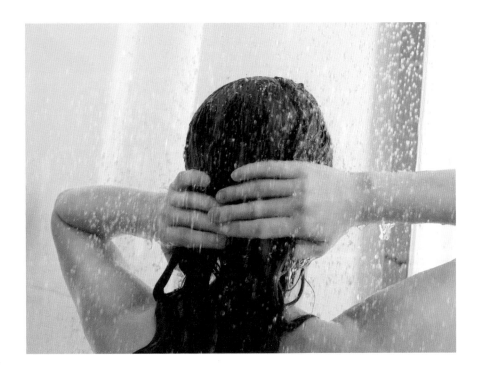

warned that it's not for everyone. It usually requires serious scalp work (scritching, preening, brushing, combing), the right kind of water, and possibly just the right kind of scalp/natural pH balance.

That said, some people do find that water on its own is the method that works best for them—even better than baking soda or another alternative cleanser. You can try to gradually transition, but don't be too distressed if the ROM is not for you. It will depend a lot on your personal makeup and what the water in your shower is like. Invest in a showerhead filter if you're really dedicated. A successful transition will take time, even if you're already shampoo-free.

Low Poo

If you're nervous of leaving shampoo behind entirely, or you're struggling to find a good shampoo alternative, seeing unhappy hair no matter what you try, give a "low-poo" product a go.

The right kind of shampoo bar makes a nice low poo. The ingredients should be simple and straightforward. J.R. Liggett Bar Shampoo, which is available in several different formulas, has similar ingredients to castile soap but is formulated as a solid bar specifically to work on your hair. A shampoo bar can be a one-stop

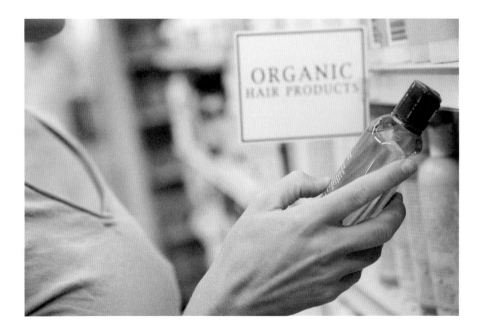

shop (no need for conditioner), which also makes it a great option for travel. Many people report happiness with the results.

Another option would be premixed shampoo and conditioner packages that resemble shampoo in most ways—minus the sulfates, parabens, etc. They are the "better brands" of shampoos, specifically formulated without ingredients the shampoo-free set wants to avoid. Peruse the products offered by Morrocco Method, 100 Percent Pure, SheaMoisture, or Desert Essence. A trip to Whole Foods or your local health store will provide even more options.

Low-poo products are nice because they're easy, mimic the traditional shampoo and condition process (if routine comforts you), and they can leave your hair looking great with minimal effort. They can be pricey though. If that's an issue for you, you could try alternating one of these low-poo options with a cheaper shampoo-free routine to get more bang for your buck. Or stick with shampoo bars—they're more cost-effective.

MY LOW-POO RECOMMENDATION

I splurge on a low-poo option once in a while to mix up my routine. I particularly enjoy the 100 Percent Pure "Healthy Scalp" line, made with burdock and neem. The products are easy to use (standard shampoo and conditioner routine), and I really like the state they leave my hair in: soft, shiny, and clean. Best of all, they assist my scalp in its annual wintertime flaky dryness battle. The products leave a nice smell behind as well (more herbal than flowery, but I enjoy it). Nothing wrong with hair smelling like hair, but sometimes it's nice to get a little fragrance without worrying about said fragrance's chemical makeup. The Healthy Scalp line contains plenty of essential oils and nourishing ingredients, which means I get all their benefits without having to buy individual bottles of each. It makes the price tag of the shampoo itself less imposing.

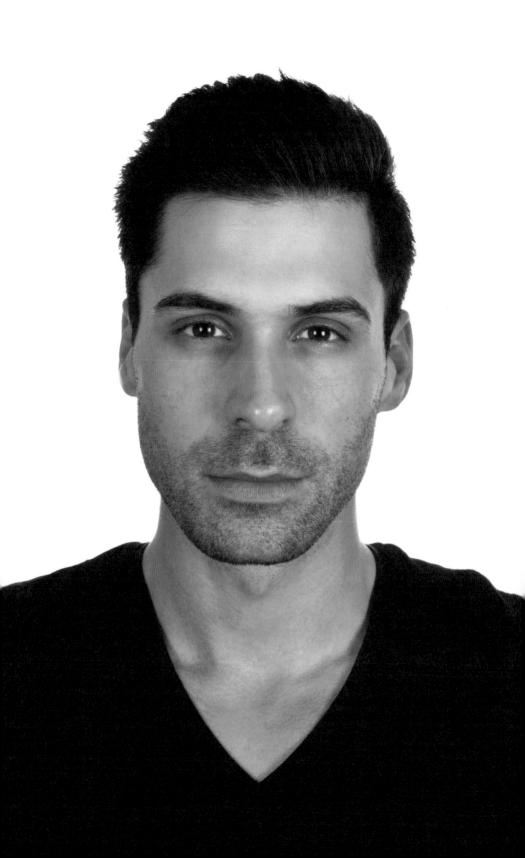

Add-Ons

Play around with herbal concoctions and essential oils to see what adds an extra spark to your locks.

For extra cleansing power, try lavender, lime flowers, or witch hazel; for dandruff, try burdock, goosegrass, or nettle; for scalp soothing and hair strength, try catmint, horsetail, or nasturtium.

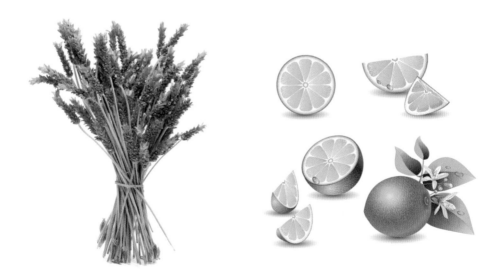

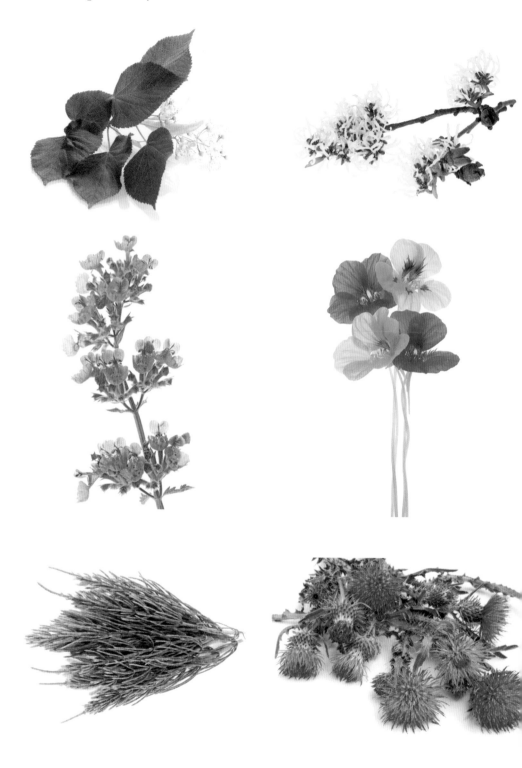

To experiment with coloring, try chamomile, marigold, or mullein to lighten, and sage, rosemary, or parsley to darken. Tea can also tweak your hair color. Darker teas, like traditional black tea, will darken, lighter teas, like green tea, will lighten, and a red tea, like hibiscus tea or rooibos, adds a scarlet sheen.

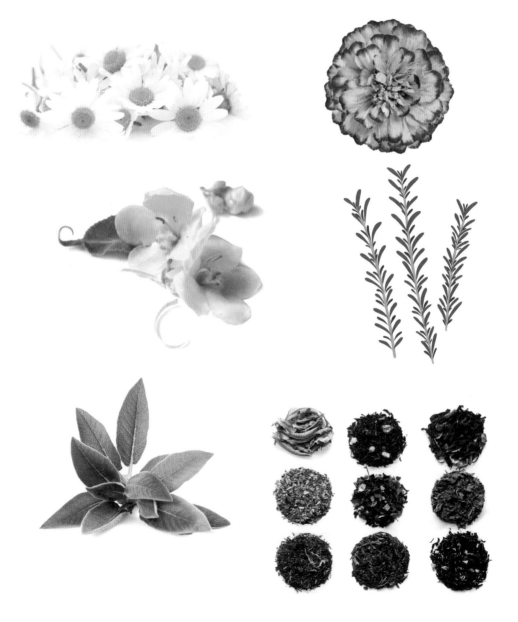

WHAT'S IN A NAME?

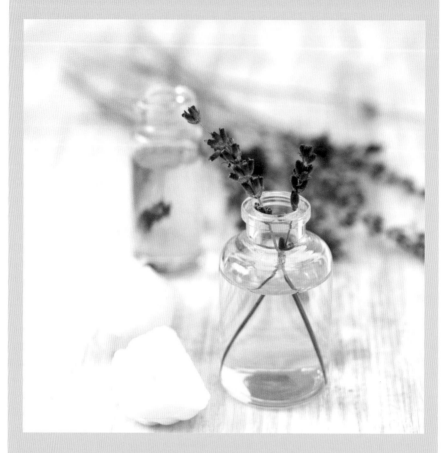

Is it a coincidence that *lavender* so closely resembles *lavare*—the Latin verb for "to wash"? Lavender may have received its name thanks to its association with washing clothes. That makes centuries of lavender in cleaning products. Why not add it to your modern routine?

Tools

Okay, now that we've talked products and ingredients, let's talk tools. First of all, particularly if you have straight or loosely wavy hair, invest in a 100 percent boar bristle brush. Nearly all of the happy shampoo-free people

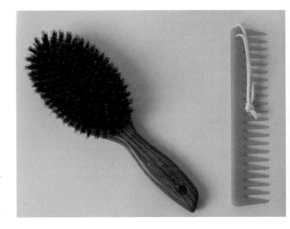

with that hair type whom I've surveyed say a "BBB" is a must. It will help distribute your scalp's natural oils, so that rather than greasy roots with dry ends, the length of your hair is shiny and soft. A denman-style brush may be better for curls than boar bristles. A wide-tooth comb can also be useful for combing and distributing products and mixtures in the shower (remember that wet hair breaks more easily, so make sure it's wide-tooth to avoid damage).

A handful of household items can also make great shampoo-free tools. A measuring cup with a spout can help you

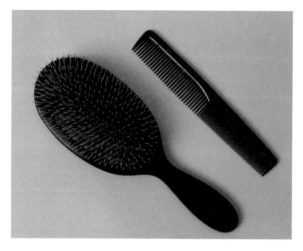

proportion your poo-free mixtures and distribute the solutions onto your head (or into another container with better controlled pour action). Spray bottles are also awesome if you are using the classic baking soda and apple cider vinegar combo. Make a mix of baking soda in one wide-nozzle spray bottle, and your vinegar mix in another. When it's hair-cleaning day, you have the mixtures easily at hand, and the spray bottle will help ensure easy and even distribution.

Another item of help? Fingernails! If you're the type to leave your nails a little long, this will help you enormously with ridding

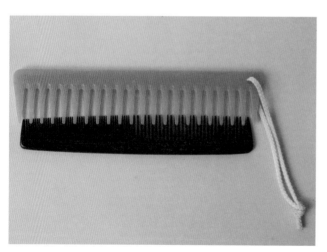

your scalp of the dry skin it no longer needs and any excess sebum that has accumulated. This process is typically called "scritching" in the no-poo sphere. It can help resolve dandruff, keep your scalp healthy, and minimize any overall ickiness. Just scratch the ick off your scalp and rinse away while in the shower. Fingernails also help with "preening"— pulling the oils in your hair down from your scalp along the length of your hair

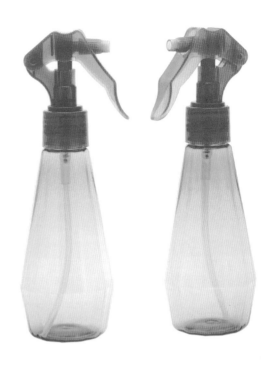

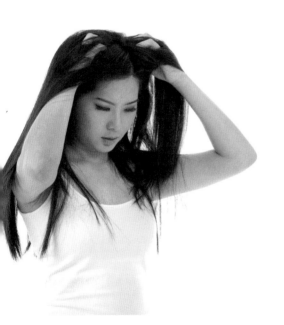

shaft, which helps protect your hair from damage and improve its moisture level and shine. It's like boar bristle brushing with your nails. If your nails are short, try the washcloth method.

WASHCLOTH METHOD

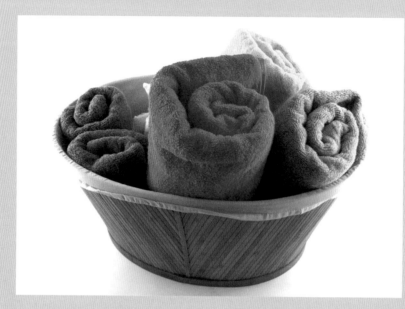

Using your boar bristle brush helps distribute healthy oils along your hair strands when hair is dry, but don't brush when wet—it will damage your hair. Luckily, you can up your healthy hair game by using a washcloth to distribute oils when hair is wet. Simply wet the cloth while in the shower and wipe down from your scalp to the ends of your hair. Try for 100 strokes on each side.

Ready? Set? Go!

Help yourself prepare for shampoo freedom by gradually tapering your use of shampoo in the months leading up to your transition.

If you shampoo every day, try skipping one day a week, then moving to every other day, then every three days, and so on. Use dry shampoo if you're having a hard time transitioning without 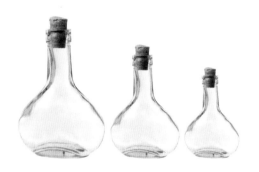 grease (the homemade kind, not the spray cans).

When you're ready to take the plunge, set your hair to tabula rasa mode. Get a trim to lose any unhealthy hair, like dry or split ends. Finally, right before your transition, do one last product detox to

get rid of the buildup left behind by styling products and certain shampoos and conditioners. Particularly products used to tamp down frizz tend to leave waxy or silicone residues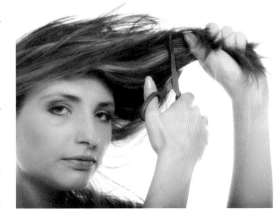

on the hair. To remove any remaining gunk, use a detoxing sulfate shampoo; a cheap drugstore one should do (as long as it has no silicones in it). Your locks should now be a blank slate.

Speaking of detoxing, your hair will likely have a crazy re-set phase while it re-regulates its sebum production in the wake of losing shampoo. You may notice this as soon as you start cutting back on your daily shampooing, or it may not kick in until later in the process, but you'll probably see at least a few bad hair days before your scalp adjusts. The transition period typically lasts from two to six weeks. Don't worry, it's temporary!—and tips for dealing with this icky phase are provided later in the book.

WHERE TO START?

Fine hair or thick, straight or curly, greasy or dry? Use your hair type and texture as an initial guide. Use the following tips to help select a "first stop" method or two.

If you have straight hair or loose waves:→Try standard BS + ACV.

If your hair is very wavy or tightly curled:→Try co-washing.

If you have fine hair:→Experiment with a henna or cassia rinse.

If you have dry hair:→Incorporate a conditioning oil.

If you have greasy hair:→Supplement with a homemade dry shampoo.

NO-POO SHOPPING LIST

If you want to give the classic "no-poo" method a shot, here's what you'll pick up at the store:

- Your alkali (e.g., baking soda, castile soap)
- Your acid (e.g., apple cider vinegar, lemon juice)

Optional add-ons:

- Two spray bottles (one for your alkali, one for your acid)
- Boar bristle brush and wide-tooth comb

That's it! Once you know how your hair responds, go back for any extras, like coconut oil, essential oils, raw honey, or aloe vera.

Once you've read through the options and selected a method, assembled an arsenal of helpful tools, and detoxed your hair to remove any products, you're ready to let the grease goblins run their course while your hair adjusts. Aim to let the transition run its course without resorting to shampoo—it can prolong the process. But don't distress if you turn to surfactants once or twice while you're figuring it all out. You'll get there!

KEEP IT SIMPLE; MAKE IT WORK

If all of the information on how to quit shampoo seems overwhelming, here's a shorter outline of how to successfully take that first trip off the diving board.

Start with a clean slate. Use a balanced cleansing and clarifying routine. Don't rinse with hard water. Remove gunk from your scalp and distribute your scalp's natural oils. Condition as your hair calls for it. Be patient. Listen to your hair. Enjoy your newfound freedom. Repeat ad infinitum.

Keep Going!

You tapered your shampoo use. You selected a method to try. You gathered your materials and tools. You even dumped out all your old shampoo bottles. (Actually, as satisfying as that would be, you may want to keep the shampoo to clean brushes and combs with. Or consider donating it to women's shelters. If those chemicals are going down the drain, someone should benefit from them first.)

Finally, you've done your first shampoo-free wash! So now what? Well, first there comes the speed bump of the detox period to surmount. Use the tips discussed in the troubleshooting section for easier navigation.

Once you've made it out of the woods, detox-wise, it still may take some time to find the ideal shampoo-free routine for you. That's okay. Be patient. If the method you tried first doesn't totally click, change it up. This could mean changing the proportions (less baking soda; more apple cider vinegar); or it could mean changing the application process (rinse the baking soda immediately; leave the apple cider vinegar on a little longer); or it could mean trying

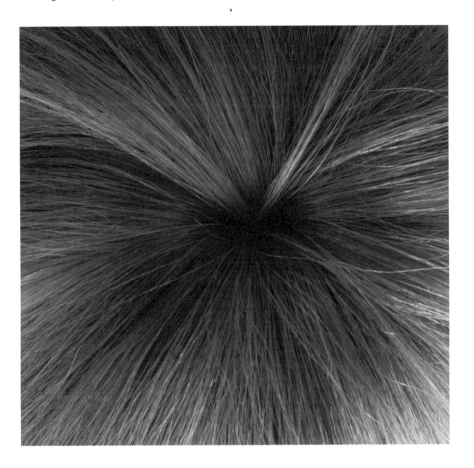

a different method (baking soda leaves hair blah; try castile soap or spend a few weeks using one of the nice conditioners we discussed).

Listing all the possible variations is not meant to discourage you. It may be that you barely notice any detoxing, and that the first method you try works wonders for you. Enumerating the options is more to let you know that if your initial results are less than ideal, that doesn't—and shouldn't—be the end of the adventure for you. Going shampoo-free can be a trial-and-error process, but once you find the routine that clicks, it will be worth it! The road may not be entirely smooth, but persistence and experimentation will help you stay the course.

SHAMPOO FREEDOM TIMELINE

Every scalp is different, but here's how you might transition to poo freedom in eight weeks.

- **Weeks one and two:** Cut back on your shampoo routine. Aim to shampoo only once a week at the end of these two weeks. If that sounds crazy, try for at least every three days. Supplement with a little dry shampoo if you like.
- **Weeks two and three:** Take the plunge and start with your no-poo alternative of choice. Be mentally prepared for the "detox" period—it will pass.
- **Weeks four and five:** You may be seeing some reduction in grease production—if not yet, soon. Experiment with your ratios, ingredients, and tools to see what works best for you.
- **Weeks six through eight:** By now, you should be well on your way to a life free from dependence on shampoo. Keep experimenting and have fun!

TRAVEL TIPS FOR HAIR CARE ON THE GO!

Leaving your daily routine behind doesn't have to mean saying goodbye to your hard-earned freedom from shampoo. These easy and portable solutions do the trick for on-the-road hair care.

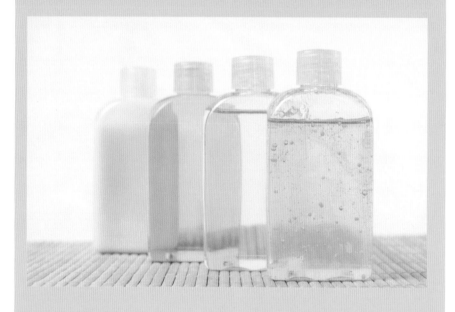

- ◆ **Co-washing.** Use the hotel conditioner, or just bring your own little bottle.
- ◆ **Shampoo bars.** A little goes a long way, and no messy liquid to worry about.
- ◆ **Dry shampoo.** Light, compact, and helps you bring less of any other materials by extending time between washes.

After-Care

Once you've nailed your routine (more or less—why not keep experimenting to see if your hair can look and feel even better?) and transitioned to shampoo freedom, you will likely be amazed at how little you need styling products you once relied on. If your hair is naturally wavy or curly, giving poo the ax will almost certainly guarantee your hair better texture and easier upkeep. Sebum is the scalp's all-in-one product solution, but there are a few more style tips to be had.

HEAT HARM

Your scalp's natural oils offer some protection against heat from a blow-dryer or flat iron if you do decide to use one. But approach with caution. Heat should be used sparingly—too much can cause damage. Shea butter and argan oil provide extra heat protection.

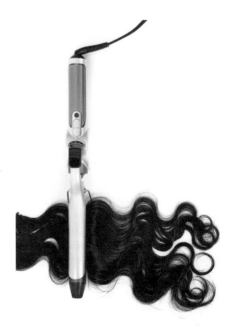

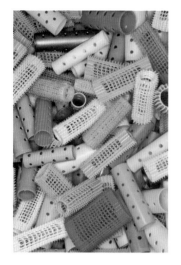

If you notice that heat is hurting your hair, take it down a notch. It's probably a good idea in general to see how low you can go. Stay away from the high setting on your blow-dryer. Try some fun heatless hairstyles like pin curls or rag curls. Experiment with different hairstyles too.

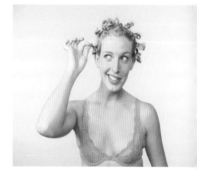

DIY STYLE

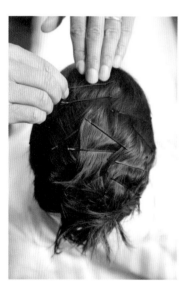

Most styling products will also contain the no-no ingredients we discussed earlier. You may find that you don't really need them now that you're shampoo-free, but if you miss your favorite hair helpers, here are a few safe and easy homemade product recipes. Make small batches so you won't need preservatives.

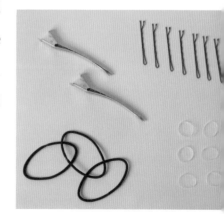

Hair Spray

Simply dissolve two teaspoons of sugar in a half cup boiling water. Let cool and then add a few drops of your favorite essential oil if you wish. The cool mixture can be placed in a bottle and sprayed as any store-bought spray.

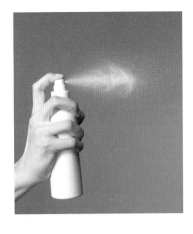

Hair Gel

Stir half a teaspoon of gelatin into one cup of hot water, fresh off a boil. Allow the mixture to set as it cools. As with the hair spray, you can mix in essential oils if you like once the mixture has reached a gel-like consistency. Or try adding a little lemon juice, aloe vera, or coconut oil to the mix.

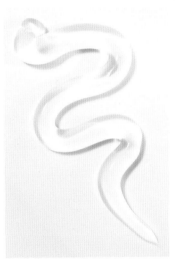

Mousse

Combine one part liquid coconut oil with two parts warm shea butter and whisk until fluffy; slowly pour in one part olive oil and mix thoroughly. Store in a lidded container. Keep away from heat and sunlight.

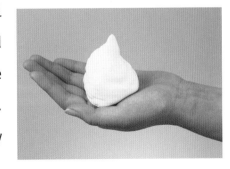

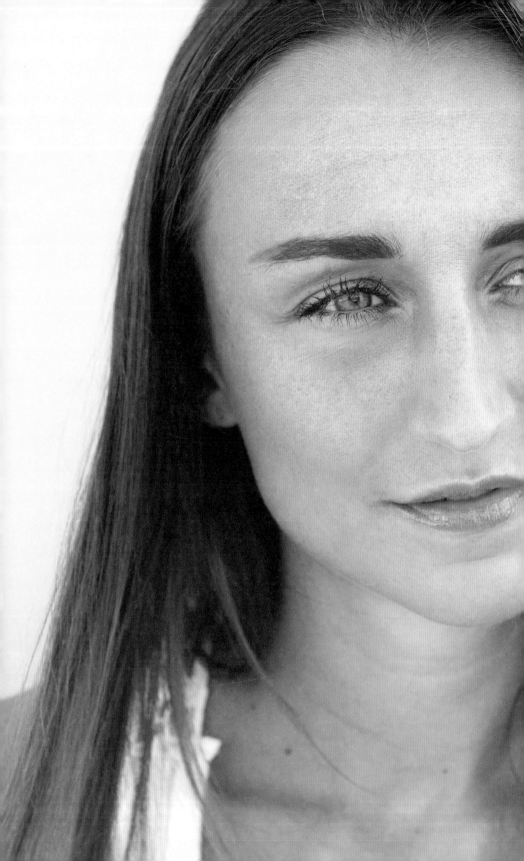

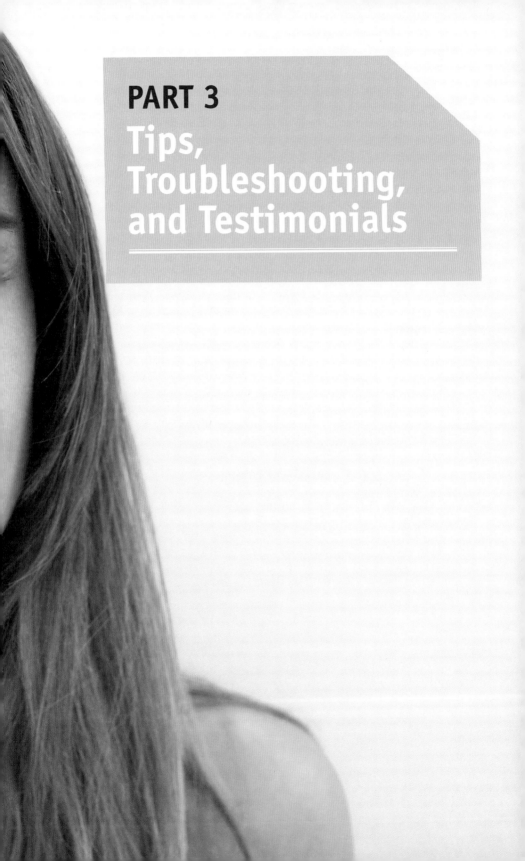

PART 3
Tips, Troubleshooting, and Testimonials

I f you're somehow still hesitating, read on to see why there's no good reason *not* to try a shampoo-free lifestyle. First, we'll tackle the common objections, issues, and questions one by one. Then we'll read joyful accounts from successful renouncers of shampoo, filled with words of wisdom and encouragement to set you on a happy path.

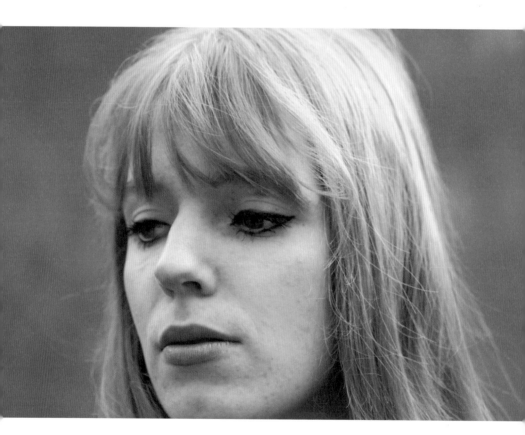

Excuses, Excuses

I've heard it all before. Guess what? Like the advertisers who once gave us Farrah follicle envy, I say to you: This too can be yours. Read on for the counters to all your "It won't work for me because . . ." prevarications.

IT'S JUST NOT RIGHT FOR MY HAIR.

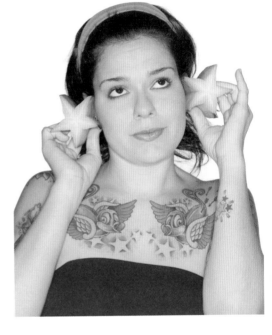

This is the number-one objection I hear from would-be converts when I extol the virtues of the sham-free lifestyle. "There's no way it could work for me—my hair just needs to be shampooed!" Your hair doesn't *need* shampoo. It may rely on shampoo at the moment, it may be too greasy when you go a while between washes, but that could be in part because you're using shampoo so often. There are shampoo alternatives for anybody's head.

I admit I had an advantage going in. I am one of those non-daily showerers that the *New York Times* promises are not disgusting (we're not!). So I already knew full well that hair could be fine without daily sudsing. I broke my too-poo habit early on thanks to the bleach, dye, bleach, tone cycle I went through from my early teens to mid-twenties (necessary first for my punk rock aesthetic and then my desire to look like a blond French New Wave star). I didn't see my natural hair color for a good ten years, and throughout that era, I washed my hair once a week at most. The bleached strands needed all the natural oil they could get. Not to mention that my hair looked scary and sad if I didn't blow-dry it (even though the heat was damaging—a vicious cycle), so I would go as long as possible between wettings to let the hair keep its shape and style.

When I finally grew it out, it was nice to lose the years of damage, but I found I could still shampoo infrequently, if a bit more often than when I was platinum blond or bright magenta.

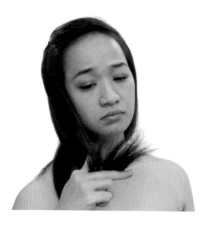

If you don't have a similar natural advantage, it does not exclude you from making the transition. You may need to taper more gradually; you may be in for a longer detox period; you may need to use your shampoo alternative more frequently at first (and maybe in general), you may want to sprinkle dry shampoo into the mix, you may never be a water-only washer, but rest assured: You can do this. See the tips in the troubleshooting section for how to make it work for whatever ails your hair.

I DON'T WANT TO BE GROSS.

Will you get gross? I shan't lie: You may be in for some grossness while your hair adjusts to its newfound freedom. Mine got disgusting! And I was never a daily shampoo user. But I also went over a month without shampooing or alternapooing *at all*. I really wanted to hit the reset button on my grease glands. Whether or not you do likewise, you'll likely see an uptick in grease while you're transitioning. Rest assured: This too shall pass.

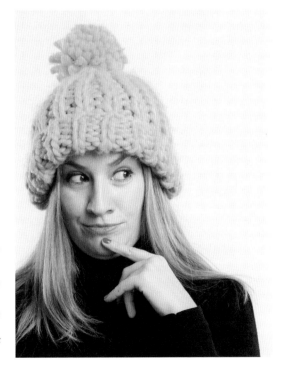

In the meantime, wear a hat. If, like me, you're lucky enough to live somewhere with a winter, that's three freebie months (seven if

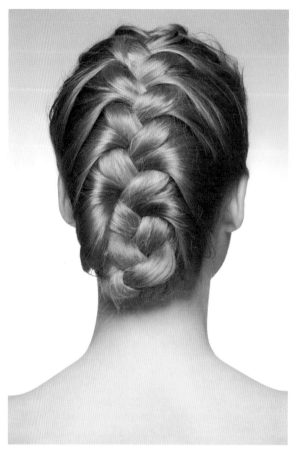

you're in the Midwest) when it's perfectly acceptable to cover your entire head with wool every time you leave the house. Also, you've always wanted to get better at the elaborate French-braiding techniques that photograph so cutely on the Internet, right? Now is your chance! Surely there is a simple trick to those crazy upside down fishtail braid buns. It's winter, so you have time to sit inside and figure it out. Once you make the transition, you will not be gross!

If winter is not an option for you (you lucky thing), there are plenty of fun updo hairstyles to try. Google is a microcosmic oyster of hairstyle tips.

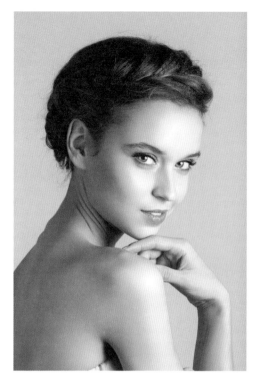
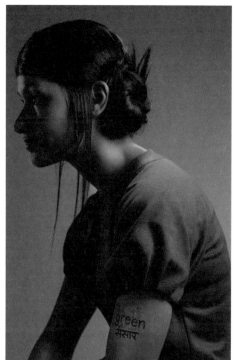
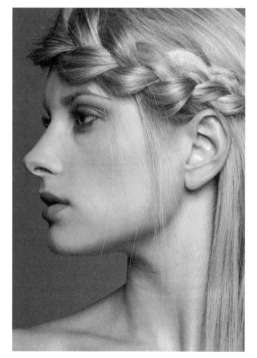
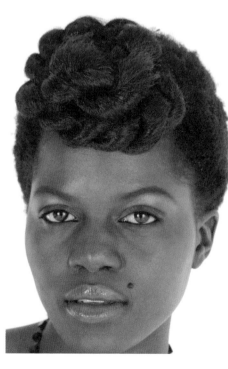

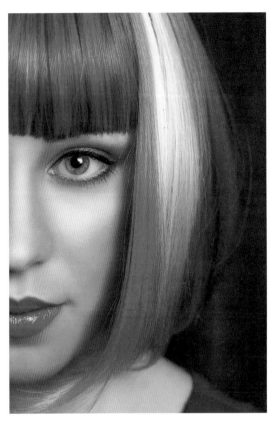

I COLOR MY HAIR.

If you dye your hair, can you still go shampoo-free? Yes. Many people with colored hair quit shampoo successfully. It may be more or less tricky depending on what shape your hair is in and what type of products you want to use. Washing hair less often will help maintain its color, obviously. It's also good to boost your hair's health in as many ways as you can to counter the damage being done by the dye. Consider switching to dyes that are easier on hair (though they may not work as well or last as long). Be aware that baking soda and castile soap (or any alkaline cleanser) may not be the best option for you because their alkalinity opens the hair's follicles, meaning the color housed there will get washed right out. If you highlight your hair, that won't be an issue though, so if you've been wanting to lighten your locks, let shampoo freedom be your catalyst.

I WORK OUT A LOT (OR A LITTLE).

What about the gym? How does one deal with all the extra sweat? It's true that letting sweat sit in your hair will not do wonders for it. But you do not need to shampoo every time you go to the gym—what a waste of products and an ordeal for your scalp.

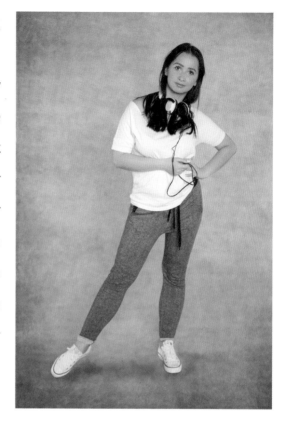

Tie your hair up during your workout and wear a large headband to help absorb some of the sweat. A simple water rinse after should do the job for most post-workout cleaning sessions. If you're still feeling gross, do a light co-wash by rubbing a bit of high-quality conditioner into the grungy areas. Dry shampoo also works—and it's easy to carry a little in your gym bag.

I SWIM OFTEN.

Chlorine can pose a problem, as can saltwater. If you're too stubborn to go the simple route of getting a swim cap (seriously,

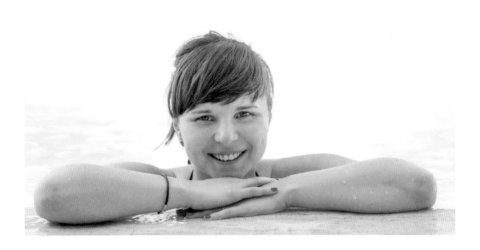

just get a swim cap!—there are some cute vintage-style ones out there), and your hair is feeling dried out, try a combo of egg yolk, olive oil, and cucumber post-swim. Don't over-egg though. Just like you don't want to eat too many eggs every day, you don't want to use too many on your hair. Or maybe your water at home has a touch too much chlorination? It might be time to shell out for a showerhead filter. Your hair and skin will reward you by getting extra beautiful.

"Okay, you've convinced me!" I hear you cry. And then, the inevitable: "But wait . . ."

SHAMPOO-FREE KIDS

If you have little ones, you may wonder whether shampoo freedom is accessible to them as well. Absolutely—perhaps even moreso the younger they are. Try water-only washing for your children from the beginning. For those times when water just

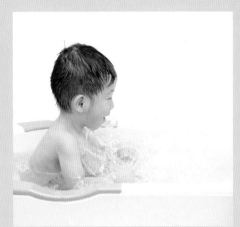

won't cut it (kids are great at finding ways to get dirty), try a healthy homemade baby shampoo, like diluted unscented castile soap. Castile soap is mild but not entirely tear-free, so rinse with caution. (Keep the vinegar and acidic rinses away from your babe—tear city!) Check the EWG's product database for safe, easy, and tear-free store-bought options.

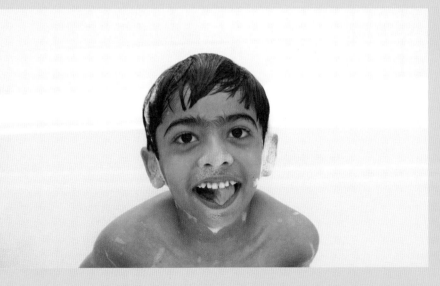

Shoot Those Troubles!

You're on the bandwagon and you've emptied your shampoo bottles down the drain like an alcoholic atoning. But the road is filled with potholes . . . You're considering going back to your plastic bottle vice. Don't worry! Here's a run-through of the most common problems, and suggested solutions for shooting them into oblivion.

GREASY HAIR

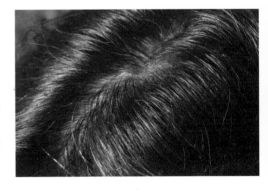

You may need a less diluted alkali. An uptick in grease is likely during the detox period, so be patient and don't go too crazy with the baking soda if you're still within the first few months. Try dry shampoo to tamp down the grease. Experiment with further diluting your vinegar mixture, or try citrus rinses. People using honey report that it sometimes leads to grease, so be aware of that as well. Egg whites on the scalp may remove excess grease if you're still struggling.

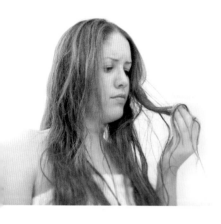

DRY HAIR

If your hair feels dry, see how low you can go. Meaning cut down on the baking soda (or whatever cleanser you're using) and cut down on the ratio of any acid you might be using. In addition, cut down on the number of washes and rinses you do. Stretch the time between washes as far as possible. Don't go crazy with the dry shampoo. Try a hot oil deep-conditioning treatment. Experiment with different conditioning methods.

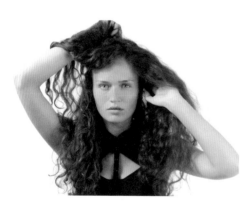

WAXY, HEAVY, OR STICKY HAIR

If your hair feels coated in waxy or sticky grime, hard water is likely the culprit. Hard water really affects your ability to use traditional "no-poo" methods successfully. Baking soda and castile soap will leave a scummy residue. Vinegar rinses can help remove some gunk, but you may still find that your hair feels like a science experiment gone wrong.

Hard water is fairly common, but if you have it, don't despair. If you have cash to burn (actually, invest), purchase a water filter or a water softener for your showerhead. More economical options: Use distilled water, or water that's been boiled (and

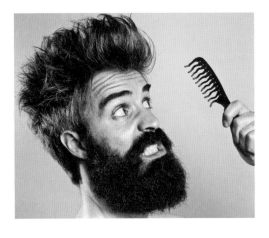

then cooled obviously!). If you're not sure whether your water is hard or soft, check out a water quality map online.

STRIPPED OR THIN HAIR

If the high pH of baking soda or castile soap followed by the low pH of ACV or another acidic rinse is a problem for your hair, the result will be thin or stripped-feeling strands.

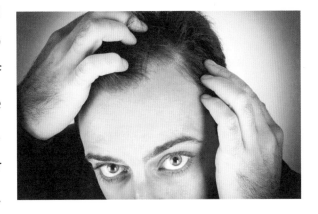

Don't fret, just switch to a more pH-balanced shampoo alternative, like aloe vera, honey, or a low-poo product. Restricting the alkali cleanser to your scalp will also help. That way, the length of the shaft won't go through the rapid pH change that is troublesome for some people. And make sure your mixes are as mild as possible.

CHALKY HAIR

Thank sebum if you're seeing chalky buildup. Like grease, an uptick in sebum is common during the detox period. Use your boar bristle brush to fight the accumulation. Some non-pooers swear every day is a must, while others find that frequent brushing

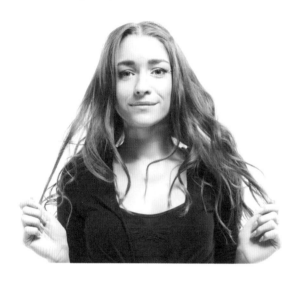

actually makes their hair greasier than desired. Find the routine that's right for you. Whatever the schedule, boar bristle brushing will make a massive difference by scraping some of the gunk off and distributing your scalp's natural oils so they don't just sit on the top of your head like a grease helmet. Pretend you are a Victorian lady (or don't, because being a lady was often a drag back then) and go for one hundred strokes before bedtime. That brush is gonna get *nasty*, particularly during your detox period, so wash *it* with some shampoo (if you have any leftover) whenever it needs it.

Plug your sink, add a healthy squirt of SLS-laced goo, and fill the basin with water. Let the brush sit in the sink for few minutes, then use a comb to loosen the gunk from the bristles. Rinse well and resume Victorian routine (only the hair-brushing part; maintain modern attitudes).

If you just cannot seem to clear the sebum hurdle even though you're following all advice to a T, here's a little secret. It's okay to cheat sometimes. One shampoo wash is not going to send you back to square one while you're still transitioning. If you feel like you've accumulated an unconquerable amount of buildup, a sulfate shampoo can help you reset. It may prolong the transition, but that's okay. Just don't make it a habit again and you'll still be walking the path to freedom.

PICKLED (STINKY) HAIR

Maybe this is obvious, but the key to not smelling like vinegar is to rinse thoroughly and/or use less vinegar. The vinegar ratio will really depend on your personal chemistry, so if you smell brined, take it down a notch. If you're secretly

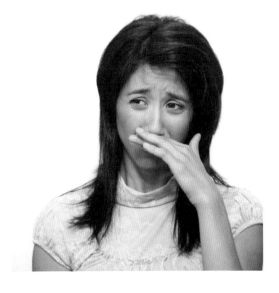

pining away for the good old scent of Spring Breeze Ocean Party Flower Goddess that your ex-shampoo imbued to your locks with its enigmatic "fragrance" blend, get some nice essential oils and put a drop or two in your vinegar rinse (or whatever your final

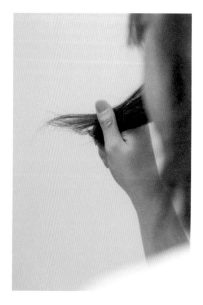

whole-head step is). Some popular scents are ylang-ylang, jasmine, rose, or carrot oil. If pickle pong just won't quit you, switch to a different acidic rinse, like a citrus-based one.

SQUEAKY HAIR

Too much alkali, friend. Lower the dose, and follow each alkaline wash with an acidic rinse.

MUSHY HAIR

Mush is the opposite problem from squeak. It means you're going too heavy on the acid, so dial it down a notch.

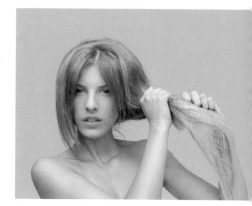

LIMP HAIR

You're likely going overboard on the moisturizer. If you're using oil, honey, or any other conditioning treatment, scale that back.

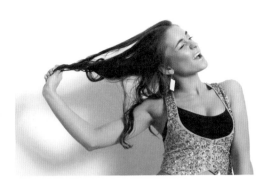

UNWANTED COLOR CHANGES

Depending on how porous your hair is, and other mystical scientific hair properties that a scientist could explain better than I can, you might find that the acidity in vinegar or lemon rinses lightens the color of your hair. If you're into it,

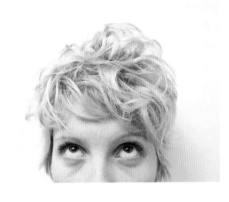

enjoy. If you're not, try honey or beer to cleanse and condition, a dark tea or coffee to counteract the lightening effect, or see if you can further dilute your rinse with the same cleaning and clarifying effect. Unwanted lightening may also occur from overuse of baking soda. If BS washes are your method of choice, aim for twice a week at most—less than once per week

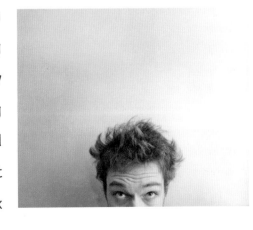

is even better. Or alternate with another cleanser so that you're using the baking soda no more than once a month.

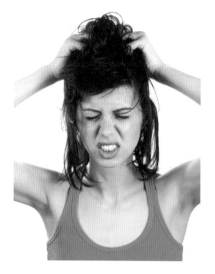

ITCHY HEAD

A few different factors could be causing your mysterious head itch.

Leaving any ingredient on too long might be the problem. Getting overzealous in your non-pooing routine might be the cause. If you were a frequent shampooer, you may be tempted to wash sans-shampoo with the same frequency. Restrain yourself. Add in some ingredients to help combat itch, like aloe, honey, or tea tree oil.

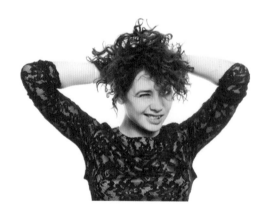

DREADED DANDRUFF

If you didn't have dandruff before you quit shampoo and are seeing flakes now, it probably means too much baking soda. Up the water ratio in your mixture and see how that goes. If success continues to elude you, reach for diluted castile soap instead. Rinse the baking soda or castile soap right away; don't allow it to sit on your head. Try doing an acidic rinse both before and after your basic wash.

If you've had dandruff *before* your transition, quitting shampoo may improve your scalp's health and lead to an overall flake reduction. But don't despair if not. Scalps are weird microcosms. Incorporate some commonly touted remedies: apple cider vinegar rinse, tea tree oil, aloe vera, or burdock. Make sure you're getting in there with that BBB or curl-friendly brush and massaging your scalp in the shower to loosen and remove flakes. Add brown sugar to your wash; the texture will help remove flakes.

Coal tar and antifungal shampoos are the more conventional option, but read up on their potential dangers first.

WAIT, NOT DANDRUFF, JUST SOME WEIRD WHITE RESIDUE?

If it's white, it's baking soda buildup. If it's grayish, then it's probably sebum buildup. (I know, ew. Hang in there!)

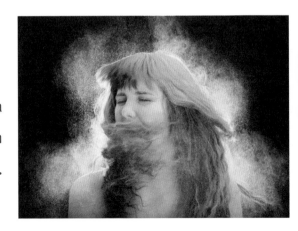

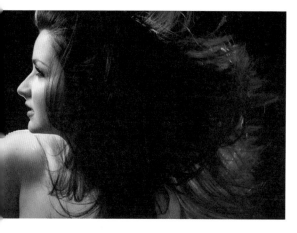

STATIC

It happens, especially in dry and/or wintry climes. Make sure your hair is properly moisturized, that you're not overdoing it on the basic washes (too much baking soda is a recipe for static), and that your hair is generally healthy (trim split ends, avoid heat).

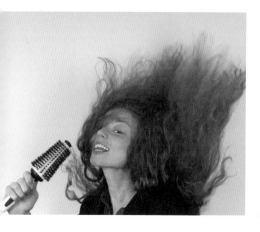

FRIZZ

Use a humectant (like honey), add some aloe, moisturize properly, stay away from too much protein, adjust your acid rinse (try a new acid, try less acid in the mixture, try leaving in on your hair for less time), and do a cool water rinse at the end of your shower.

HAIRY HAIR

Hair will be hair. Meaning, everyone's hair has its wants and its needs, and those are influenced by myriad factors, known and unknown. The demands of hair differ from one person to the next; they differ one day to the next on the very same scalp. The real key to troubleshooting? Above all, adapt to your hair. Every morning when you wake up, ask your locks what they're looking for. Some days it'll be a wash; some days your whole head is good to go. Some days hair wants extra moisture and conditioning. Some days it wants brushing. You don't need to do everything the same every day; routines can be freeing—they eliminate the energy of assessment and decision-making—but of course they're also limiting. Shampoo freedom means freeing yourself from those limits and taking a day-by-day approach to happier hair.

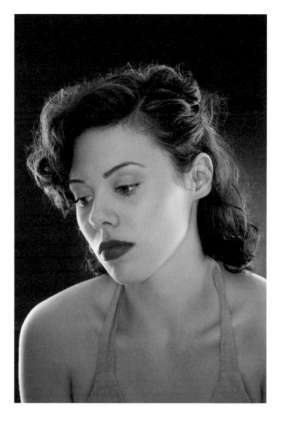

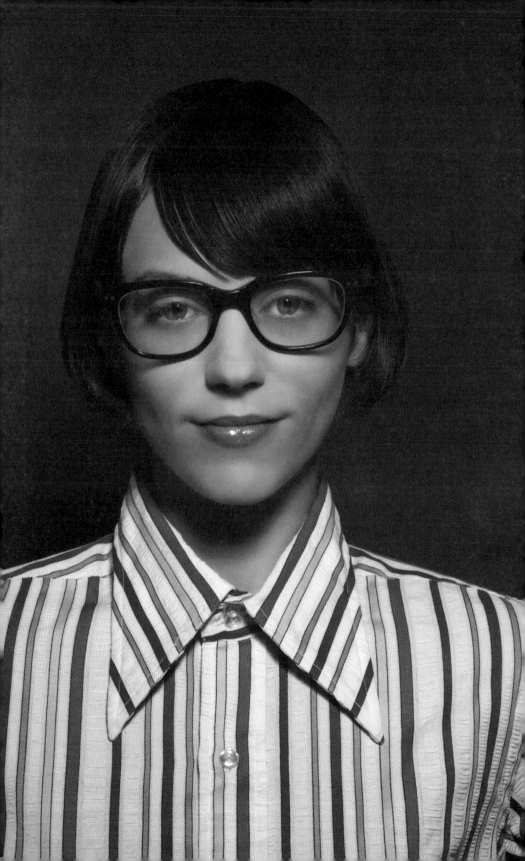

Testimonials

Enough about problems. Time for some inspiration. In this section, hear from folks who've made it! That is, they've triumphantly attained freedom from shampoo. The shampoo-free lifestyle can be practiced by anyone, no matter what type of hair you have. From some of the Internet's finest shampoo-free writers to everyday enthusiasts of healthy beauty routines, this section is all about success stories. Their insights will help your find yours!

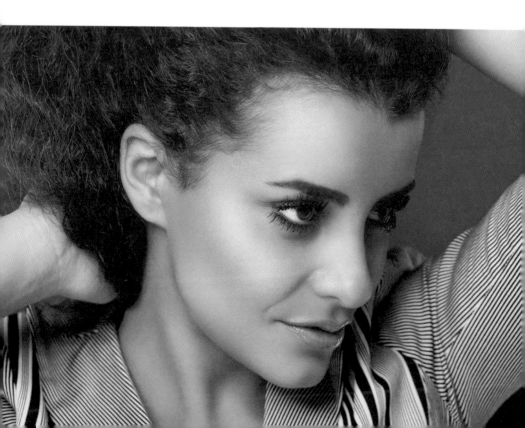

LAUREN'S STORY

Lauren O'Neal brought her tale of shampoo freedom to the masses with her wonderful series of advice articles published on the *Hairpin*. Who could resist a piece titled "How to Quit Shampoo Without Becoming Disgusting"? Turns out, pretty much nobody—Lauren's posts are among the most popular in the history of the site. Her writing is equal parts wit and wisdom.

HAIR TYPE AND TEXTURE:

Thin and very fine. Clips, pins, elastics slide right out.

HOW LONG SHAMPOO-FREE:

Since the beginning of 2011, so coming up on four years. (Four more years! Four more years!)

WHY DID YOU GO SHAMPOO-FREE?

Actually, my original motivation was my skin, not my hair. Standard conditioners would give me breakouts wherever my hair touched my skin on my face, shoulders, and upper back. I had also just been vaguely unhappy with my hair—it didn't look *bad*, but it didn't look *good* either. So I decided to try quitting shampoo and see what happened, and then I was unexpectedly zapped into an alternate dimension where everything's the same except there's no such thing as bad hair days.

HOW HAVE YOU BENEFITED FROM BEING SHAMPOO-FREE?

Well, number one, my hair looks awesome, which gives me such a confidence boost in day-to-day life. It's really nice that I only have to worry about my hair once a week and that it stays clean for several days, so I don't go from Clean Human to Swamp Beast overnight. My inner hippie is also very satisfied that I use less plastic and introduce fewer harmful chemicals into the environment. ("Chemicals" is a fraught term, but you know what I mean.)

WHAT IS YOUR TYPICAL HAIR-CARE ROUTINE?

Every five to seven days, I wash it with baking soda and then with apple cider vinegar. I just keep a bottle of each in the shower, diluted with water. I play around with the dilution level a lot, but I'm currently using one part baking soda/ACV to two parts water.

HAVE YOU ENCOUNTERED ANY DIFFICULTIES OR OBSTACLES?

The detox period at the beginning is gross, but it's temporary. Also, there are a lot of people on the Internet who think I'm delusional and dirty, but people on the Internet also think that lizard people control the government and that racial slurs are a cool way to express yourself. People who see me in person don't think these things, obviously, because they can see for themselves they're not true.

DID YOU EXPERIENCE A "DETOX" PERIOD?

Yes! I went about four or five weeks just washing my hair with water and nothing else. (I bet you'd detox just as well with two weeks, though.) It was gross, but not *that* gross, because it's only really your scalp that gets oily, and the rest of your hair stays more or less the same. Your hair just looks kind of dirty for a few weeks, it's not the end of the world. Tips to get through it: Brush your hair often; it scrapes a lot of the grease from your scalp. Clean your brush often; it's full of scalp grease. Headbands and hats are also helpful.

WHAT DO YOU DO WHEN YOU TRAVEL?

If I'm traveling for fewer than five days, I just wash my hair with baking soda and ACV the day I leave and then don't worry about it for the rest of the trip. If I'm traveling for more than five days, I bring my diluted bottles of baking soda and ACV. I used to use bottles that were easy to accidentally open via suitcase-jostling, and that's the story of how I arrived in Hawaii with all my clothes and books soaked with vinegar. I had even put them in a plastic freezer bag, but the freezer bag had a tiny hole in it! Now I use different bottles, and intact freezer bags.

DO YOU STYLE YOUR HAIR OR USE STYLING PRODUCTS?

I do some minimal styling. After I shower, I flip my hair over and blow-dry it in sections with a finger diffuser for about ten minutes, which makes my hair look wavy and not just oddly messy. On windy days (which is almost every day in San Francisco), I use a homemade "sea-salt spray," which I'm putting in quotes because I actually make it out of Epsom salt and aloe vera. Then the wind gives me "beachy waves" instead of "some tangles that are piled on top of each other in an attempt to simulate human hair." I've also made a mostly functional hair gel out of flax seeds, but I don't really find it to be worth the effort.

WHAT IS THE MOST IMPORTANT PIECE OF GUIDANCE YOU WOULD OFFER SOMEONE WHO WANTS TO GO SHAMPOO-FREE FOR THE FIRST TIME?

Experiment with the level of dilution on the baking soda and ACV until you find the one that works best for you. It seems to vary a LOT from person to person. Also make sure to rinse the vinegar out thoroughly so you don't smell like a pickle jar, *no matter how much you love pickles.*

BIO

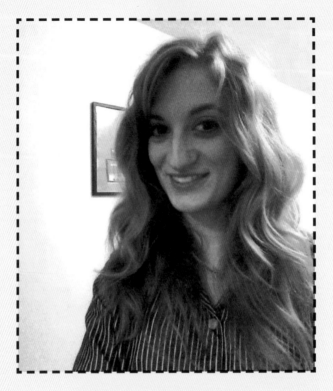

Lauren O'Neal is a freelance writer and editor in San Francisco. Her writing has appeared in publications like *Slate*, the *New Inquiry*, and the *LA Review of Books*. She is the former assistant editor of the *Rumpus* and is currently an associate editor at *Midnight Breakfast*.

ALISHA'S STORY

Alisha Cole is the force behind Motown Girl, an informative website "dedicated to helping readers learn how to style and manage naturally curly/kinky hair at home." Alisha's educational work has inspired and assisted scores of natural hair-care enthusiasts, and the Motown Girl site provides an abundance of healthy hair intel.

HAIR TYPE AND TEXTURE:

I describe my hair type as a mixture of mostly 4A with sections of 3C. The 4A sections are soft with tight coils and the 3C sections have a looser curl. Sometimes hair products respond differently to the various sections; overall it has been quite a trial-and-error process learning how to deal with the different hair textures.

HOW LONG SHAMPOO-FREE:

Over a decade!

WHY DID YOU GO SHAMPOO-FREE?

When I used traditional shampoos too often it made my hair hard and tangled after a while. Even after moisturizing and deep conditioning, at times my hair became brittle. While I never experienced hair breakage, my hair back then had less elasticity and more frizziness compared to my hair currently.

WHAT IS YOUR TYPICAL HAIR-CARE ROUTINE?

About once a week, I normally use castile soap followed by a deep-conditioning treatment. As part of my process, I use a high-quality deep conditioner, add extra virgin olive oil, and leave it on my hair for thirty to sixty minutes. During the week, I occasionally "wash" my hair with water only, and others times I will co-wash with a light conditioner.

I do not use regular shampoo. I prefer to use castile soap and sometimes I use glycerin or oil-based soap bars. Recently, I've been experimenting with do-it-yourself shampoo recipes. It has been fun playing around with various essential and fragrance oils, etc.

After cleansing and conditioning my hair, I add a little cold-pressed virgin coconut oil, put into two or four braids, and let it set overnight. The next day I unravel the braids and will either put my hair into a high bun or leave it half up and half down. This hairstyle is called a braid-out. The braids stretch my hair out while leaving a slight kinky wavy pattern that I love. Putting in more braids equals a tighter, more defined wave pattern and less braids equals a looser wave.

HAVE YOU ENCOUNTERED ANY DIFFICULTIES OR OBSTACLES?

I've worn my hair natural for almost fourteen years now—during this time I've had *a lot* of trials and errors! At this point, I'm completely comfortable and confident with my hair routine. However, early on in my hair journey, I found myself in a hair product frenzy, as I was always buying and trying something new and I spent a lot of money in the process. However, I have been no- or low-pooing since 2002 and I've found that my hair has needed less hair products as the years have gone by.

WHAT DO YOU DO WHEN YOU TRAVEL?

When traveling, I do not require many items for my hair, but I make sure I pack travel-sized hair conditioner, hair gel, and hair tools, such as bobby pins, headbands, and a wide-tooth comb. I almost always work out in a hotel gym, so I usually will co-wash with my leave-in conditioner and style as normal.

DO YOU STYLE YOUR HAIR OR USE STYLING PRODUCTS?

Yes, I style my own hair every day. The only styling products I use are a leave-in conditioner and hair gel to slick my hair back into a bun or ponytail. I do not use heat to style my hair, nor do I use any chemicals (color, texturizers, etc.).

DO YOU HAVE ANY OTHER HEALTHY HAIR TIPS?

Apple cider vinegar rinses are great to get rid of product buildup, can soften the hair, and get rid of an itchy scalp and dandruff. I typically use one tablespoon of Bragg's ACV to sixteen ounces of filtered water, rinse through my hair, massage it into my hair and scalp for about two minutes, squeeze the excess out, and style as usual. I find the scent dissipates after a few minutes.

To detangle my coils, I use a wide-tooth comb and/or a denman brush. When my hair is wet and soaked with conditioner, I detangle starting from the ends and work my way up to the roots. These tools help the process go a lot faster and smoother, and the conditioner provides a much needed "slip," which helps to reduce breakage.

I also use raw and unprocessed honey on my hair as a hair mask during the warmer-weather months. Honey is a humectant as it helps to draw in moisture, which allows added hydration for the hair. It provides my hair with added softness and natural sheen.

Coconut oil is great on my hair after a co-wash. I use it as a sealant to help lock in moisture, smooth out frizz, and to set my hair when wearing braid-outs. I've tried all kinds of oils on my hair, but once I tried coconut oil I was hooked!

WHAT IS THE MOST IMPORTANT PIECE OF GUIDANCE YOU WOULD OFFER SOMEONE WHO WANTS TO GO SHAMPOO-FREE FOR THE FIRST TIME?

To those thinking about the "no poo" routine, I would first recommend to keep an open mind. Your hair will not smell and it's not uncleanly. No-pooing simply cleans without stripping the hair of its own natural oils (sebum).

When washing your hair with conditioner, you will not get the soapsuds like when using SLS (sodium lauryl sulfate) based products. Keep in mind, you will still get the desired results with clean hair, just minus the suds. This was something that took me a little time to get used to myself.

Secondly, you can make the transition from shampooing with regular conditioners or "low pooing" with sulfate-free shampoos, as these products are typically more gentle on your hair.

Lastly, don't expect miracles in a week. A no-poo hair routine will take some trial and error. Depending on your lifestyle and preferences, you will need to figure out a routine for you. Take photos of your hair prior to starting and during. I recommend giving your hair approximately one month to see if this routine works for you or not.

BIO

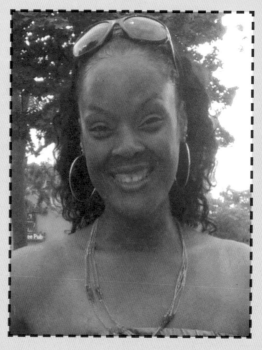

Alisha Cole is the founder of MotownGirl.com, a website offering homemade hair recipes, step-by-step hair styling tips, and a popular "MG Spotlight" series, where readers from all over the world submit personalized Q&A profiles to be featured. Motown Girl has been online and adding new content since May 2001.

HEATHER'S STORY

Heather, aka Babs of the blog Babyslime, is a true fount of shampoo-free wisdom. Her blog offers countless tips, explanations, and words of encouragement, and is a must-bookmark for any poo-free newbies. Her advice is extraordinarily comprehensive and equally as useful.

HAIR TYPE AND TEXTURE:

Up until very recently, my hair was moderately thick, straight, and smooth. It's thinned out quite a bit now that I've entered menopause though.

HOW LONG SHAMPOO-FREE:

Just about ten years now. My eldest is eleven, so she's been shampoo-free almost her whole life, and my youngest two children (eight and three) have never had anything else on their hair.

WHY DID YOU GO SHAMPOO-FREE?

I have severe chemical and scent allergies/sensitivities, so living a more natural lifestyle was a no-brainer for my family from

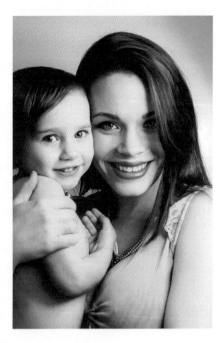

the get-go, and there were only a handful of shampoos that I could handle without feeling ill anyway. I first discovered the method through whispers and scattered posts on "natural living" Internet forums, almost all of which were followed by rave reviews of how well the process worked. Something that drew me to it in particular was discussion of how it improved hair's natural volume, seeing as it eliminated the conditioner-buildup problem of traditional shampoo/conditioner use; my hair has never been naturally voluminous and I've always wanted it to be. Even after my first try at "no poo," I could see a huge difference in my hair's volume and texture (so shiny and silky!) and I was sold!

HOW HAVE YOU BENEFITED FROM BEING SHAMPOO-FREE?

Well, the compliments sure are nice! I get complimented on how nice my hair looks by strangers on a regular basis and that never happened to me as a shampoo user. My hair is always amazing after a wash, and I honestly didn't even know it could get so soft. The only drawback is that I can't stop touching it . . . which means I end up rubbing all my hand oils into it and have to wash it again in another three to four days.

WHAT IS YOUR TYPICAL HAIR-CARE ROUTINE?

I use a slightly higher than typical dilution of baking soda (about 1.5–2 tablespoons of it per 1.5 cups of water) and a slightly lower one for ACV (about 0.75 tablespoons per cup of water) because I find it works best on my hair, and after I'm out of the shower, I use a bit of argan oil on the bottom third of my hair, most concentrated on the ends. I don't brush it out until it's dry to avoid breakage, but honestly I find that all it needs is just a bit of finger-combing to be tangle free! The ACV rinse plus a touch of oil automatically detangles it, even when it's still pretty wet. Once dry I'll run a paddle brush through, and maybe a boar bristle brush to get the oils well distributed.

HAVE YOU ENCOUNTERED ANY DIFFICULTIES OR OBSTACLES?

Hormonal changes are a big one! When I'm pregnant, and now that I'm in menopause, the texture and oil production of my hair changes dramatically. I find that my whole routine is thrown for a loop and it takes a while to figure out what my hair needs. But other than that, I've had a pretty easy time of it! My husband started getting dandruff when he moved here to Canada from the very dry Mojave Desert in Southern California, and once we switched to no poo, it went down significantly but didn't disappear completely. He found that doing a white vinegar rinse about once a week or so worked very well to keep it in check.

DID YOU EXPERIENCE A "DETOX" PERIOD?

I don't recall my detox being all that dramatic, but I do remember that it lasted a while. I used a bit of the cornstarch trick to absorb some oil (a little cornstarch brushed through your scalp can help absorb it, then brush it through/out with a bristled brush), but for the most part, I kept it braided to help hide some of the oiliness until it was all done. This was easier since at the time I lived way up north in the middle of a pretty awful winter (about -35° to -45C° on a daily basis), so having your hair covered up was no big deal.

I was a heavy-duty conditioner user prior to giving it up, and I think my best tips would be on easing back your conditioner use for at least a week or two prior to starting your detox to ease it through. I also found that it helped initially to wash my hair every three days until my hair was back to its natural state, and then go with what it needed at that point (usually once every four to six days, except during pregnancy/menopause).

WHAT DO YOU DO WHEN YOU TRAVEL?

If I'm traveling locally, or staying with friends and family, I either take two little travel bottles with me with pre-made mixes, or just borrow from my friends' pantry! Almost everyone has baking soda in their cupboard, and most have ACV. When I'm traveling for business and going across the country or out of it completely, I generally just bring an undiluted travel bottle of ACV (so I can dilute it myself when needed) and then ask the hotel kitchen for baking soda or pick some up at a grocery store. I've always been able to get a little cup from the hotel kitchen though; they always have it on hand for baking.

Only once did I end up caught without anything after getting in to my hotel very late (and in desperate need of a shower), and ended up using the hotel body soap to wash my hair. Fortunately they didn't have hard water, so it didn't leave any buildup, and I didn't have to go through detox again from going back to shampoo . . . but I wouldn't recommend it!

DO YOU STYLE YOUR HAIR OR USE STYLING PRODUCTS?

Not typically; I'm a mom of three young kids and don't exactly go out too much with the little free time I have, so I'm not big on products and fancy styling. I only do my hair up nice when I'm working large events (I'm a professional photographer), and then I find that a touch of hair spray or gel is all that's needed. I tend to gravitate to the more organic/natural end of the spectrum anyway (see above reasons about sensitivities) and I've had no problems with their usage and no poo.

DO YOU HAVE ANY OTHER HEALTHY HAIR TIPS?

Definitely argan oil! It's lovely, especially for split ends or damaged/dyed areas. I have a chunk of hair bleached and dyed and I use it most on that area to keep it moisturized and fight off the damage from the bleach, and it's really wonderful stuff. If argan oil is too pricey (or not available), coconut oil is the next-best bet.

A good-quality boar bristle brush is also a must. I hear the Pearson brand is the best for this, but it'll run you about $85 . . . which is just a bit more than I'm willing to spend on a hairbrush. Thankfully, most other decent-quality boar bristles only run about $20 to $30, and they are worth the purchase if you can get one (best for straight or wavy hair; you'll probably find it just angers your curly hair).

I've heard amazing things about kaolin clay treatments for dry hair, especially if you're a person of color who wears their hair natural. Kinky hair benefits amazingly from it! Frizzy hair can too. I haven't tried it yet myself, but it's on my list of luxuries.

WHAT IS THE MOST IMPORTANT PIECE OF GUIDANCE YOU WOULD OFFER SOMEONE WHO WANTS TO GO SHAMPOO-FREE FOR THE FIRST TIME?

Patience! The detox can seem gross for some people, especially previously heavy users, but it's absolutely worth it to wait and see how lovely your hair can be!

Also, be flexible and willing to experiment once your hair is out of detox! Play with the dilutions a bit and see what your magic mix is. If you have very hard water and are having trouble finding a good balance that doesn't leave your hair still feeling greasy, try using distilled/nursery water specifically to rinse your hair with when you wash it: It's usually only a buck or two for a gallon and if you only use it twice a week just to rinse out your mixes, it's totally worth the small hassle. I've heard from quite a few people that this made all the difference when they were close to giving up.

BIO

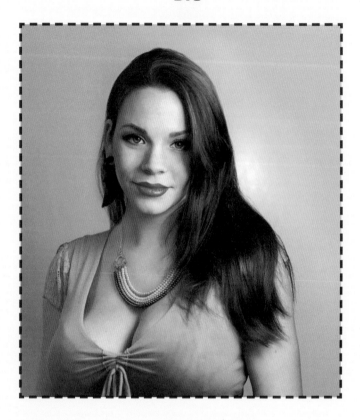

Heather is a writer, photographer, mother of four, and wife of twelve years. She has been blogging since 1999 on subjects ranging from disability and disease to birth and motherhood to sexuality and activism. Find her online at Babyslime-blog. com.

SONNET'S STORY

Sonnet Lauberth is the voice behind In Sonnet's Kitchen, a seasonal cooking blog featuring original recipes, beautiful food photography, health and wellness tips, and DIY home and beauty remedies. Sonnet's work is guaranteed to make you excited about healthy living. (It will also make you very hungry!)

HAIR TYPE AND TEXTURE:

Medium texture, slightly wavy.

HOW LONG SHAMPOO-FREE:

On and off for five years. I was pretty steady with being shampoo-free for three years, then fell off the wagon for a bit.

WHY DID YOU GO SHAMPOO-FREE?

I had heard about the "no poo" method and although I thought it sounded weird at first, I was intrigued. It seemed like a healthier, more sustainable, and affordable option than using expensive shampoos and hair-care products.

HOW HAVE YOU BENEFITED FROM BEING SHAMPOO-FREE?

In my experience, baking soda and vinegar actually give my hair a much better texture than shampoo! When I used shampoo and conditioner my hair was always fine and limp, but now it has more body and volume.

WHAT IS YOUR TYPICAL HAIR-CARE ROUTINE?

I mix one part baking soda with four parts water and apply it to the roots of my hair. I rub this into my scalp for a minute then rinse with warm water. Then I mix one part white vinegar with four parts water and run this through my hair, followed by rinsing with cool water. I found that rinsing with cool water seals the hair cuticle and leaves my hair shinier. I use this every two to three days and use a homemade "dry shampoo" on the other days if my roots feel a little greasy. Most days I let my hair air-dry, but in cooler weather, I follow this with a hair dryer and sometimes a flat iron.

HAVE YOU ENCOUNTERED ANY DIFFICULTIES OR OBSTACLES?

Although the leftover vinegar smell in hair is very slight, it can be noticeable if someone is close to your hair. This usually isn't a problem in general, but if you're dating someone who doesn't like the smell of vinegar, it can be a bit of a challenge. I found that adding essential oils to the vinegar rinse helps to reduce the smell if it's bothersome.

DID YOU EXPERIENCE A "DETOX" PERIOD?

I never experienced a detox period and, in fact, I found my hair to be less greasy than it was when I was using shampoo and conditioner. However, on the days when I don't use my baking soda and vinegar method, I use a homemade "dry shampoo" of arrowroot powder mixed with cocoa powder (since I have darker hair). This works well for absorbing any oiliness and I usually recommend it to folks who are struggling with their hair.

WHAT DO YOU DO WHEN YOU TRAVEL?

I usually bring a small container of baking soda and then a travel-sized bottle of vinegar so I can use this method even while traveling.

DO YOU STYLE YOUR HAIR OR USE STYLING PRODUCTS?

Occasionally I'll use a homemade "hair spray" of sugar water (this helps to hold hair in place), but usually my hair doesn't need it.

WHAT IS THE MOST IMPORTANT PIECE OF GUIDANCE YOU WOULD OFFER SOMEONE WHO WANTS TO GO SHAMPOO-FREE FOR THE FIRST TIME?

Don't be afraid to try it. If it doesn't work for you, you can always go back, but definitely try to keep an open mind. You might be surprised at the results!

BIO

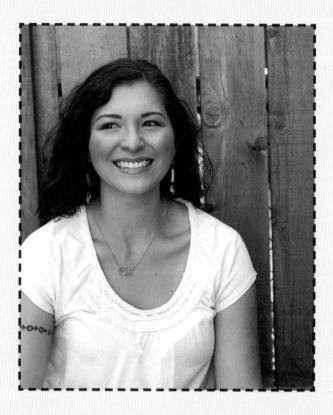

Sonnet Lauberth is a certified holistic health coach, cookbook author, blogger, and writer on a mission to help people create fresh food that nourishes their body and life. Find her work at InSonnetsKitchen.com.

ERICA'S STORY

Erica Abunda is a queen of crafts and all-around aesthetic maven. Her blog Spines and Seams chronicles her journey into the land of shampoo freedom, and you'll definitely want to check out her gorgeous handmade jewelry as well.

HAIR TYPE AND TEXTURE:

It is a bit coarse, long, thick, and a bit wavy.

HOW LONG SHAMPOO-FREE:

More than a year now.

WHY DID YOU GO SHAMPOO-FREE?

I always got that weird smell from my scalp even right after a shower no matter how much I washed my hair and scalp. My hair also got very weak and dry from all the shampooing.

HOW HAVE YOU BENEFITED FROM BEING SHAMPOO-FREE?

I got rid of that weird scalp smell! I rarely get split ends now and people have noticed that my hair looks healthier, more

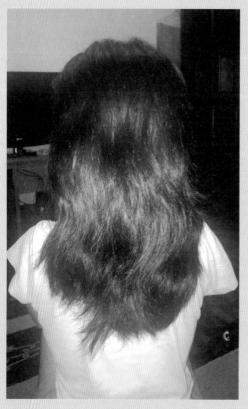 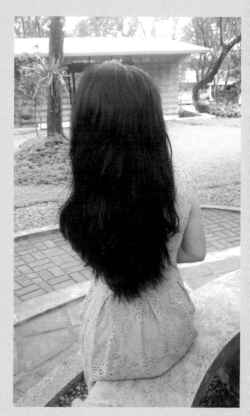

Before   **After**

shiny, and even more black, if that makes sense. Of course, I've saved money now that I only buy ACV every other month. I haven't even bought a new box of baking soda ever since I started.

WHAT IS YOUR TYPICAL HAIR-CARE ROUTINE?

Right now, I comb through my dry hair with a wide-tooth comb before a shower. I rinse my (wet) scalp with about a teaspoon baking soda in about two cups of water (I eyeball every measurement now). I scrub that in until it feels slippery, rinse that out with water, immediately mix a half-cup of ACV to two cups of water, and apply the rinse to my ends and also to my scalp. I leave that in for about five minutes and rinse everything out thoroughly with cold water. I do this when my scalp feels gross with dead skin/dandruff; if my scalp just feels oily after a few days, I just rinse out with the ACV rinse.

I squeeze out extra water with my hands, and then with a towel, then apply a small amount of coconut oil to the ends of my hair. Once my hair dries completely, which takes a lot of time, I comb through it again with a wide-tooth comb and then use a boar bristle brush every other day.

HAVE YOU ENCOUNTERED ANY DIFFICULTIES OR OBSTACLES?

I am working for an international non-governmental organization right now, which requires me to be out on the field for several days a week. This also means I'm under the sun and sweating a lot. I make sure I wash my hair during the weekends, so I can just wash my hair with water during the extra sweaty days.

DID YOU EXPERIENCE A "DETOX" PERIOD?

I don't think so . . . Before I went completely no-poo, I was using sulfate-free shampoos and silicone-free conditioners, so I guess that helped with the transition.

WHAT DO YOU DO WHEN YOU TRAVEL?

I avoid washing my hair when I travel, but I just wash with water if necessary.

DO YOU STYLE YOUR HAIR OR USE STYLING PRODUCTS?

No. I don't feel the need to, really. My hair looks great on its own. I almost always have it up in a bun when I'm working, anyway.

DO YOU HAVE ANY OTHER HEALTHY HAIR TIPS?

A boar bristle brush and coconut oil are musts for me.

WHAT IS THE MOST IMPORTANT PIECE OF GUIDANCE YOU WOULD OFFER SOMEONE WHO WANTS TO GO SHAMPOO-FREE FOR THE FIRST TIME?

Don't be afraid: It's almost always not as gross when you first start out. Just tough it out and your hair and scalp will love you.

BIO

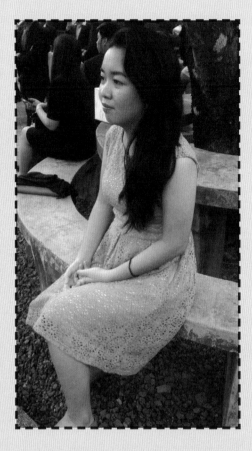

Erica Abunda is an avid writer and creative mastermind living and working in Manila. Visit her blog Spines and Seams at SpinesandSeams.wordpress.com.

LIZ'S STORY

Elizabeth Lark-Riley is a wonder-woman of the performing arts scene and all-around fan of banning unnecessary muck from our health, beauty, and daily routines. She's happily shampoo-free and encourages everyone to give it a shot!

HAIR TYPE AND TEXTURE:

I'd say my hair is thin . . . but I have a lot of it. Straight but holds curl well.

HOW LONG SHAMPOO-FREE:

A little over three years now.

WHY DID YOU GO SHAMPOO-FREE?

My friend Louise turned me onto the idea of eliminating harmful chemicals from every aspect of my life. Going shampoo-free was one of many changes I made in my personal and household-care routines to get rid of all the gross chemicals I had been living with.

HOW HAVE YOU BENEFITED FROM BEING SHAMPOO-FREE?

Being shampoo-free is *way* cheaper than using traditional shampoo and conditioner. Not only because the substitutions I'm using are less expensive but also because the poo-free alternatives don't strip my hair or gunk it up, so I don't have to wash my hair nearly as often. I went from shampooing daily to no-poo washing once every three or four days.

WHAT IS YOUR TYPICAL HAIR-CARE ROUTINE?

Every three or four days, I brush my hair and really massage my scalp with a natural bristle brush. Then I wet my hair and scrub my scalp with Dr. Bonner's liquid soap (it actually foams pretty nicely). After that I rinse thoroughly and then pour a big bowl of apple cider vinegar and water (about two tablespoons vinegar to roughly eight cups of water) over my head. Then I comb through my hair with a wide-tooth comb while still in the shower. I leave the vinegar mixture on my hair for about five minutes while I shave my legs or wash my face. Then I rinse with cold water. When my hair is still wet (before I even towel it off), I rub the tiniest amount of coconut oil on the very ends. Then I towel off and let it air-dry. I usually do this before bed and it's beautiful in the morning.

HAVE YOU ENCOUNTERED ANY DIFFICULTIES OR OBSTACLES?

It took a while to find the right routine (I tried baking soda and other things before hitting on the one that works for me), and it took a while for my hair to acclimate. But I'd say the biggest challenge is that it takes a little more prep than just hopping in the shower. I have to prepare the vinegar rinse and make sure my comb is in the shower. Sometimes the extra effort required makes me a little lazy about washing my hair . . . so then I get creative with updos and other ways of disguising dirty hair. Also, the no-poo method doesn't work so well with blow-drying . . . If I try to blow-dry rather than air-dry it sometimes ends up looking a little oily on the ends. But that's fine since blow-drying is damaging anyway.

DID YOU EXPERIENCE A "DETOX" PERIOD?

Yes, there was about a month-long detox period. My hair didn't know what to do and it was pretty greasy. I wore my hair up a lot.

WHAT DO YOU DO WHEN YOU TRAVEL?

I bring a small container of Dr. Bonner's and a small container of vinegar. I mix the vinegar with water wherever I am.

DO YOU STYLE YOUR HAIR OR USE STYLING PRODUCTS?

Only bobby pins.

DO YOU HAVE ANY OTHER HEALTHY HAIR TIPS?

A good natural bristle brush is essential. I brush my hair every night to help distribute the natural oils in my scalp to the ends of my hair. Also every month or so (if I remember), I do a coconut oil mask. To do this, I get my hair damp and then rub a generous amount of coconut oil on my scalp and throughout my hair to the ends. I leave this on for at least an hour (sometimes overnight . . . the longer the better) and then wash as described above. It's soooooooo soft afterward.

WHAT IS THE MOST IMPORTANT PIECE OF GUIDANCE YOU WOULD OFFER SOMEONE WHO WANTS TO GO SHAMPOO-FREE FOR THE FIRST TIME?

Patience and persistence!

BIO

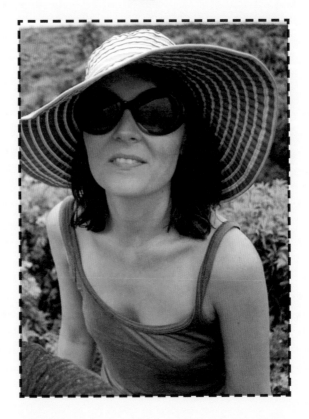

Elizabeth Lark-Riley is and actor, director, producer, and arts administrator who has lived, worked, and studied in New Orleans, New York, Chicago, and Chongqing, among other locales. She is the co-founder and executive producer of miR theater (MadeinRockledge.org), which creates and presents original performance works in Rockledge, Florida.

Conclusion

Congratulations! You are well on your way now to liberating yourself from shampoo's hold, and are sure to soon reach general hair guru excellence. Enjoy the experience. Experiment. Have fun. Listen to your hair. It will thank you!

This book is designed to cover all the basics, but so much more information is available online to assist you as you get into the nitty-gritty. Well-researched articles, message boards, forums,

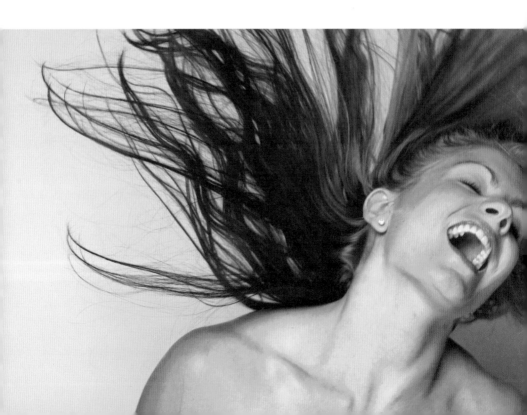

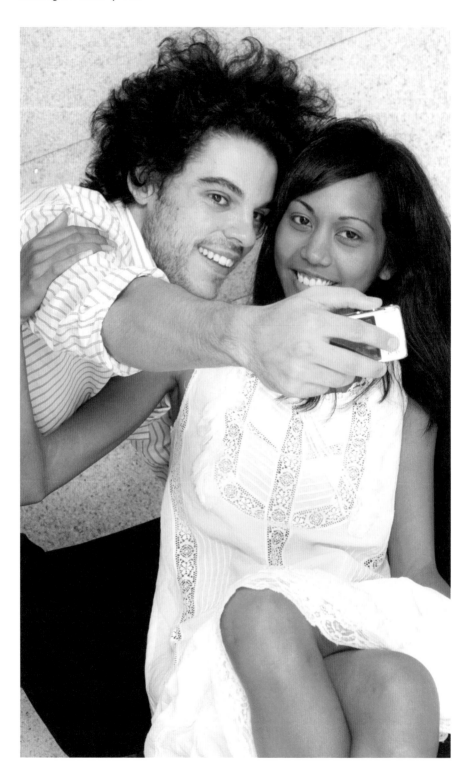

blogs, tips, videos, and all-around helpfulness—it's all just a click away. In addition to the stand-out work from the ladies featured in the testimonials section (all of it a must-read!), some of the most informative shampoo-free resources I know of are Curly Nikki's website, Crunchy Betty's blog, the Black Girl with Long Hair site, Alex Raye's Almost Exactly blog, and the work of the teams at MamásLatinas, and those behind the DevaCurl line of products and NaturallyCurly.com. Don't hesitate to take advantage of what's out there.

Thanks for taking the time to learn about the world of shampoo freedom, and best of luck on your journey to healthy, happy hair!

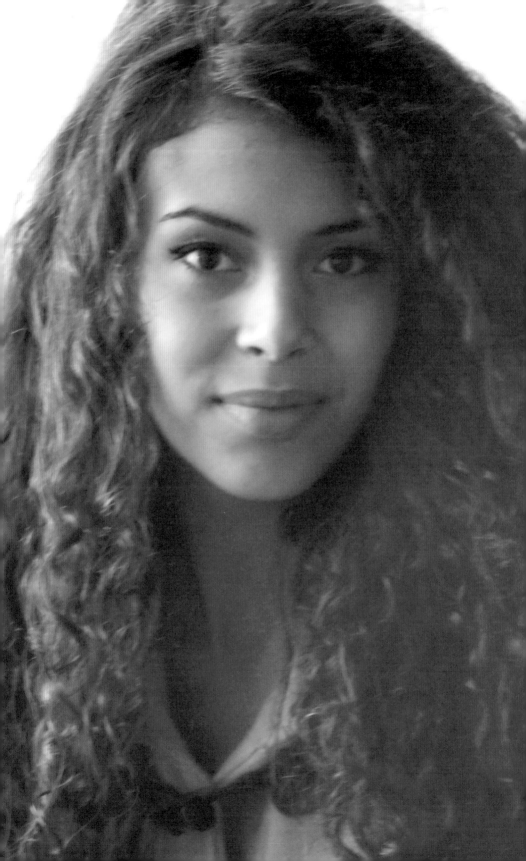

Acknowledgments

Extensive and expansive thanks are due to Jennifer McCartney, lighthouse and spark; to Rebeca Olguín, creative spirit with a mind for design; and to Sarah Grieb and Erin Albrecht, for their singularity of sight. SG, you're the reason I ditched sham. Thanks for blazing the trail.

Lauren, Alisha, Heather, Sonnet, Erica, and Liz, thank you for showing us all how it can be done and fun. This book is better because you're in it.

Thanks also to Patrick MacGowan, unwavering enthusiast (for the product, if not always the process); JDQ, general celebrant; Daniel Lupo, true eagle eye; "V in Brooklyn"; and to all the friends who encouraged, suggested, listened, or experimented.

And, of course, I owe all of it all to PMVB.

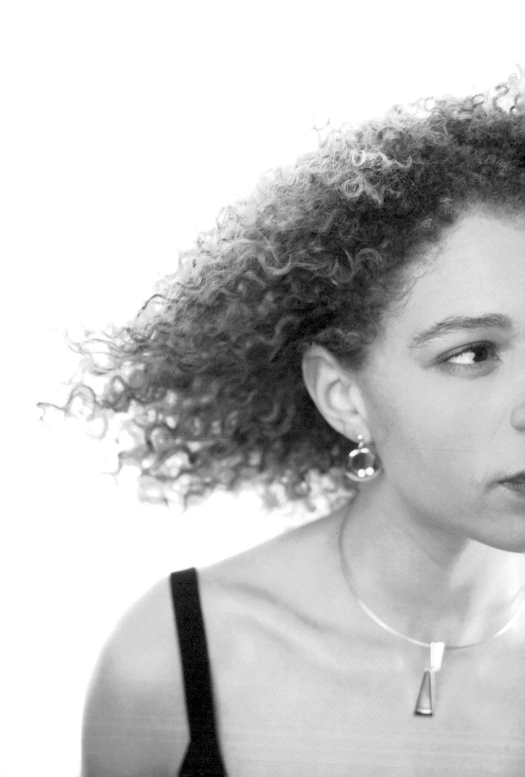

About the Author

Savannah Born is a writer and editor living in Brooklyn, NY. She enjoys information, evaluation, organization, argumentation, world-viewing, words, and wine. With the exception of a few last-resort slip-ups (which she blames on funky water, ocean overexposure, and the limitations of suitcase-life), she has been shampoo-free for nearly two years and plans to keep it that way.

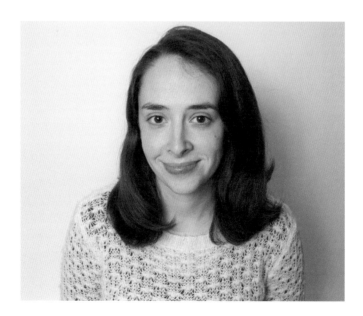